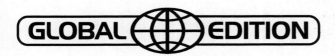
GLOBAL EDITION

Statistics Basics

A RESOURCE GUIDE FOR HEALTHCARE MANAGERS

Jennifer K. Cowel, RN, MHSA

Introduction adapted by Rainer U. Hilgenfeld, MD, MPH
Foreword by Leanne Laidler, BN, MBA
Reviewed by Maureen Connors Potter, BSN, MSN

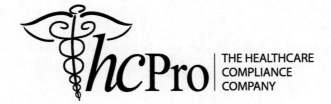

hcPro   THE HEALTHCARE
COMPLIANCE
COMPANY

Statistics Basics: A Resource Guide for Healthcare Managers, Global Edition is published by HCPro, Inc.

ISBN: 978-1-60146-188-9

HCPro, Inc., provides information resources for the healthcare industry.

HCPro, Inc., is not affiliated in any way with the Joint Commission International (JCI), or The Joint Commission, which owns the JCAHO and Joint Commission trademarks.

Jennifer K. Cowel, RN, MHSA, Author

Rainer U. Hilgenfeld, MD, MPH, Contributing Author

Leanne Laidler, BN, MBA, Contributing Author

Maureen Connors Potter, BSN, MSN, Reviewer

Mary Stevens, Senior Managing Editor

Brian Driscoll, Executive Editor

John Novack, Group Publisher

Dianne Barrett, Cover Designer

Dennis Ludvino, Layout Artist

Karin Holmes, Proofreader

Darren Kelly, Books Production Supervisor

Susan Darbyshire, Art Director

Claire Cloutier, Production Manager

Jean St. Pierre, Director of Operations

Advice given is general. Readers should consult professional counsel for specific legal, ethical, or clinical questions.

Arrangements can be made for quantity discounts. For more information, contact:

HCPro, Inc.

P.O. Box 1168

Marblehead, MA 01945 USA

Telephone: 800/650-6787 or 781/639-1872

Fax: 781/639-2982

E-mail: *customerservice@hcpro.com*

Visit HCPro at its World Wide Web sites: *www.hcpro.com/global* and *www.hcmarketplace.com*

03/2008
21382

Contents

Contents

List of figures

About the author

Jennifer K. Cowel, RN, MHSA

Jennifer K. Cowel, RN, MHSA, is a vice president with Patton Healthcare Consulting, LLC. Prior to joining Patton Healthcare Consulting, Ms. Cowel held a variety of leadership and management roles during her tenure of more than 17 years with The Joint Commission. She was a surveyor for the hospital program and served as the surveyor representative on The Joint Commission's Standards Improvement Initiative. Prior to that, she was The Joint Commission's director of service operations, responsible for authoring and managing the annual operational expense budget. She participated in the implementation and testing of *Shared Visions—New Pathways*® and the creation of management tools and a paperless tracking system for the 10,000 accreditation reports produced each year.

In addition, Ms. Cowel worked in The Joint Commission's *ORYX* program, managed the introduction of Core Measures into Joint Commission-accredited hospitals, and integrated core measures into the accreditation process. She developed and directed the launch of The Joint Commission's Network Accreditation Program, and directed the Agenda for Change initiative, which streamlined standards and redesigned accreditation survey.

Prior to joining The Joint Commission, Ms. Cowel was a senior consultant in the healthcare practice of Anderson Consulting in Chicago, Illinois, U.S.A., and she worked as a nurse on the Renal Transplant Unit at Indiana University Hospital in Indianapolis, Indiana, U.S.A.

Ms. Cowel received a bachelor of science degree in nursing from Indiana University in Indianapolis and a master's degree in health services administration from the University of Michigan in Ann Arbor, Michigan, U.S.A.

Maureen Connors Potter, BSN, MSN

Maureen Connors Potter, BSN, MSN, is Vice President for International Services at The Greeley Company, HCPro's consulting and education division, focusing on patient safety improvement in hospitals worldwide. She leads the development and distribution of publications, information, education, training, and consulting to the global market.

Prior to joining HCPro, Ms. Connors Potter was executive director of accreditation at the Joint Commission International (JCI) from December 2004 to December 2006. During that time, she was responsible for JCI accreditation products and operations, including development of standards and survey processes, marketing, business development, and relationships with international clients, organizations, governments, and accrediting bodies. She directed international accreditation products and services in the hospitals, ambulatory care, clinical laboratory, disease management, home care, and long term care programs, as well as management, hiring, and staff development for corporate office and field staff members.

She was The Joint Commission's executive director of disease-specific care from January 2002 to December 2004. In that role, she managed the start up, development, and implementation of business strategies and activities associated with disease management programs, and directed the product enhancement process to improve the value proposition of certification products.

Foreword

by Leanne Laidler, BN, MBA

As a nurse and manager/leader in healthcare, I am pleased that this book is available to support healthcare workers in understanding the basics of statistics methodology and how to apply statistics in the healthcare setting for quality improvement.

In my early days as a director of nursing, I employed a researcher to run compulsory basics-in-statistics courses for nurses and nonclinical managers and for case managers. To me, an understanding of statistics is a mandatory competency for any manager or clinician. As clinicians and/or managers, we have a professional obligation to practice on an evidence base and to analyze and improve the care and service we provide.

Understanding the basics of statistics enables you to form questions, structure a project, gather data, and then interpret these data. This is the essence of evidence-based practice and quality improvement. Evidence can be obtained in the form of research published in the literature, and an understanding of basic statistics enables the professional to critically analyze and consider these results. When measuring our own organization's performance, we may want to compare our practice outcomes with those already published. This can demonstrate that our outcomes are either comparable to those published in evidence, or they may be stronger or weaker. If the organization's results are weaker, then an argument for practice change has been established.

In healthcare settings, it is commonly the case that, in order to bring about practice improvement change, members of the multidisciplinary team need to be engaged and convinced. If you are delivering an argument based on "I think" or "I feel" or "I want," typically these will fail to compel the team. If you produce data as evidence with practice comparison outcomes, then you will have the team's attention and can build an argument for change that is more likely to succeed.

In my career, I have had the opportunity with my teams to utilize statistics in many different ways. One example has been in the evaluation of case management initiatives in the acute care setting. Statistical analysis was utilized in a range of longitudinal outcome studies comparing and measuring the impact of care. We used the Medical Outcomes Trust's short forms 12 and 36 (survey tools to measure a baseline of quality of life, then gauge improvement after healthcare interventions, such as surgery or disease management programs). We also used a variety of clinical data generated from clinical pathways, and other selected validated tools appropriate to the patient population group.

The studies utilized the preadmission phase and baseline measures using the short forms and functional measures prior to intervention. Data was collected as per study design while in the hospital and then postdischarge data at predetermined time frames after care intervention. For example, postcardiac surgery patients were followed at one month, three months, six months, and 12 months. Arthroscopy patients were followed at one week, three weeks, and six weeks. Patient satisfaction with the process of care was also measured.

We conducted studies to discover what our outcomes were, to understand the range of normal healing and return to function, and to use this knowledge to improve aspects of care, including redesigning pathways, and with more surety

 Statistics Basics, Global Edition

educating patients prior to their hospital stay. For example, with evidence, we could say 95 percent of patients have full return to function at six weeks post-intervention—pain is controlled, swelling subsided, and energy returned. Before conducting these types of outcome studies, we did not really know what the impact of our care on patients was and where our educational and operational deficits were.

The data would be presented at the organization's patient care review committee (a multidisciplinary meeting) and at the medical advisory and nursing councils. It was also used at specialty peer review meetings. Some of these studies were published but most were used internally for quality improvement purposes only. This was more due to our own resource limitations at the time. The projects supported the organization's commitment to continuity of care and provided data for surveyors when reaccreditation occurred.

Statistics methodology is also very important when measuring staff and patient satisfaction. To achieve a data safety index that is strong and reliable for management decision-making, it is essential to understand what the appropriate sample size is. Whether you are conducting this in-house or outsourcing to enable benchmark comparison data, as a healthcare professional, you must be able to interrogate the product, understand the methodology, and identify the strengths or weaknesses of what is being offered to you.

Healthcare is a competitive, challenging, and dynamic environment. As healthcare leaders, we have a professional obligation to understand what we do and the effect we have on our patients. We also need to understand how both our staff and patients perceive us. This is important for retention of our scarce and greatest asset—people—and for recruiting to the organization.

Understanding what our patients think of us is important from a care provider perspective, but is also essential in order to communicate this to our third-party payers.

None of this can be achieved without an understanding of basic statistics, so I hope you enjoy exploring the concepts contained in this book.

Leanne Laidler, BN, MBA, is group vice president of nursing and learning at ParkwayHealth Ltd., a hospital group in Asia. She is responsible for nursing and learning across the four divisions of ParkwayHealth in Singapore, North Asia, South Asia, and Southeast Asia. Ms. Laidler is a frequent speaker at conferences related to case management and quality.

Introduction

Adapted by Rainer U. Hilgenfeld, MD, MPH

"You can't manage what you don't measure!"

These words were supposedly uttered more than 200 years ago by Admiral Horatio Nelson, victor of the battle of Trafalgar. We do not quite know what he measured, but we do know that he won this and many other sea battles, so he must have done something right.

But how does this translate to the healthcare sector and its managers? Medicine has not been spared from measurement. Mortality rates have been measured as early as in the discovery of sepsis. However, in recent years, performance measurement with well-defined process and outcome indicators has gained enormous popularity in healthcare systems all over the world. Many underlying reasons can be named, including:

- Countering any perceived and or real decrease in quality as a result of cost reductions

- Increasing public accountability through measurement and public reporting

- Creating fiscal accountability through pay for reporting and pay for performance

- Increasing awareness that accreditation and performance measures are truly complementary concepts

Many countries have established some form of mandatory reporting of healthcare performance data, sometimes with public reporting, and sometimes without.

Although it has often been argued that such efforts inevitably lead to unwanted effects—including forging data and adverse selection of high-risk patients—the collection, analysis, and reporting of performance data are here to stay and require healthcare professionals to understand the basics of data analysis. In fact, there are now international databases where hospitals can anonymously compare their own performance to comparable hospitals in their country or abroad with regard to certain indicators, such as surgical site infections, patient falls, and others.

Unfortunately, many healthcare professionals do not perceive statistics or data analysis as central to their mission but as hindering their true purpose—the provision of good and comprehensive care to patients. Healthcare is too often still perceived as an "art," impenetrable by data-driven management tools. Too frequently, we in healthcare still rely on methods developed when scientific medicine and the modern hospitals emerged almost 200 years ago.

Given the competitiveness of healthcare markets all over the world, the collection, aggregation, and analysis of meaningful performance data can mean the difference between success and failure, not to mention the legitimate interest of stakeholders, including health ministries, payers, insurers, and—last but not least—the public, in increasing transparency and accountability.

Therefore, it is essential that healthcare professionals develop a basic understanding of statistics and their application. A fundamental knowledge of statistics will enable them to assess the performance of their own hospital

         Statistics Basics, Global Edition

with a critical eye and understand the messages that the performance reports convey based on the statistical methods used. And that's just the beginning.

Statistics and data analysis are an integral part of healthcare today, and like it or not, their role in all aspects of healthcare will only expand in the future. Those who can generate meaningful data, interpret it, and present it to audiences at every level will have a competitive edge when it comes to surviving in the arenas of reimbursement, public reporting, pay-for-performance programs, and even patient satisfaction.

Valid statistics can also aid in demonstrating compliance with accreditation standards, assist with pinpointing areas of care requiring improvement, and play a direct role in patient safety and quality improvement efforts.

Four trends may warrant specific attention:

- Increasingly, payers are linking payments and reimbursements to outcome. In some countries, such as the United Kingdom and the United States, reimbursement is, in part, already based on performance and will be increasingly performance-based in the future. The introduction of diagnosis-related groups in many countries has set the foundation for an increased focus on the transparency of hospitals' performance in general.

- While focusing mainly on the structure and processes of a healthcare organization, international accreditation systems are increasingly aware of the need of measurement to assess processes more continuously and focus on outcomes.

- Statistics can help you to distinguish the areas that really need improvement from those where a lack of quality is only perceived—a common problem in the healthcare sector, where, in any hospital at any time, various committees will work on topics that do not really represent major problems for the organization. Here, statistics will help you to quantify the problem.

- Using valid data also helps you to provide feedback to colleagues about their work. This can help to motivate them and create a better basis for teamwork within your organization.

This book will help you figure out what information you need, collect the necessary data, and then present your data and talk about it like a pro. However, this book will not make you a master statistician—that could take years, and it's not your job! This book also will not delve into the mathematical underpinnings of statistical theory: A working knowledge of statistics does not require mastery of complex mathematics and formulas.

The book will give you the practical knowledge, tools, and expertise necessary to collect good statistics, analyze them, display them in the best way, and make valid assumptions and improvements based on the data. It will give you the confidence to speak with authority and complete basic statistical analysis with certainty.

This book will also demonstrate that you don't need sophisticated statistical software or mathematical experts for the vast majority of what you are asked to do—you can do it with a little guidance and some how-to tips, plus the tools in this book, as well as those that you already have in your organization, such as Excel spreadsheet software.

How to use this book

This book will give you a solid understanding of statistics, the basics of:

- Study planning
- Data collection
- Data presentation
- Data analysis

Beginners can use the concepts and exercises in this book to gain a working knowledge of statistics and analysis, then apply this knowledge to gather and use meaningful statistics for any task. The focus is on statistics-related issues that you might encounter in your work, or that are required by accreditation standards, pay for performance, or other external improvement initiatives.

This book starts at the beginning: what statistics are. Chapter 1 defines common statistical terms and concepts and explains these elements' roles in quality data gathering. Later chapters focus on planning which data to collect in order to gather quality information. Each chapter includes common problems you may encounter, along with possible solutions.

You'll also find an assortment of checklists, charts, sample data, and step-by-step instructions for accomplishing a wide range of statistics-related activities. Common computer software has put statistics at the fingertips of folks like you and me, and this book will help you conquer any Excel anxiety you might have.

Who will benefit from reading this book?

Performance improvement coordinators who have been presented with loads of data, charts, and reports from their performance improvement committee and the departments that they must now support.

Staff leaders of departments that are embarking on a performance improvement initiative—your staff have been collecting data. Now you want to know what to do with it!

Nurse managers in a new specialty, who are expected to collect data for insurers, payers, associations, or hospital leadership. These groups are demanding ever-increasing amounts of data, and you have been asked to improve or explain the numbers. Where do you start?

Any healthcare professional interested in the increasing influence that data will have on a facility's bottom line. Your reimbursement may be diminished if audits reveal problems with submitted data, and you don't want reimbursement to be penalized because of poor data.

Hospital leaders hoping to stay ahead of pay-for-performance issues. Potential customers may already be trying to assess your facility's quality. Perhaps they're looking you up on various Internet sites or are reading your organization's quality report or other information.

Good or bad, right or wrong, statistics are painting a picture of your organization's quality. If customers perceive a problem with your treatment of cardiac patients or pneumonia care, they might think twice about sending a loved one to your facility. You want to make sure your facility or system is ready as pay for performance and other measures are phased in.

So let's get started!

Rainer U. Hilgenfeld, MD, MPH, is a board-certified internist with a degree in public health from the Johns Hopkins University School of Public Health in Baltimore, Maryland, U.S.A. He is intimately familiar with outcome measurement, having introduced and supported the International Quality Indicator Project

 Statistics Basics, Global Edition

from the Maryland Hospital Association (www.internationalqip.com) in Germany, Italy, Luxembourg, Switzerland, and Asia. Having also prepared numerous hospitals for Joint Commission International accreditation and having worked as a World Health Organization expert on quality management in hospitals, he has extensive experience with both measurement and accreditation—a crucial asset given the emerging alignment of both.

Getting started

What is covered in this chapter:

- Words and concepts used in statistics

- The steps in the statistics cycle

- How the statistics cycle is part of the plan, do, check, act (PDCA) cycle

- Things to keep in mind during the plan phase

Let's start at the very beginning: Just what is statistics?

If you look up the word "statistics" online or in a dictionary, you are likely to find a definition that's similar to this one: "a branch of mathematics dealing with the collection, analysis, interpretation, and presentation of masses of numerical data."[1]

To state it simply, statistics is the use of numbers to describe our world, and we use statistics every day to help us make informed decisions.

Statistics are used in healthcare and, in particular, quality improvement projects, to:

- Assess problems
- Guide and implement policy changes
- Measure performance

In all likelihood, you've been asked to gather statistics for at least one of these purposes. Whether you're using statistics to demonstrate compliance with Joint Commission International (JCI) standards, to show your hospital's exemplary record of care to an outside healthcare reporting organization, or to measure for an internal performance improvement (PI) initiative, you'll start from the same assumption. That assumption is that future outcomes will not change over time if you don't make changes in the process.

You're probably going to be charged with using statistics to predict future trends and analyze the effect that a variable (part of the process) has on the outcome.

This chapter starts with the fundamentals. First, it will explain the basic terms and fundamental concepts at the core of statistics. These are the words and ideas that are included in almost all healthcare statistics projects.

Perhaps the most important statistical concept to understand is that statistics is a process, a cycle of measurement and analysis. This chapter will show you how to get a project started using the familiar Plan-Do-Study (or Check)-Act cycle of PI. Your organization probably already uses this cycle, widely known as PDSA or PDCA, to plan and execute a wide variety of projects.

Correct use of the statistics process will not only help your organization's improvement efforts and decision-making, but will also enable you to demonstrate compliance with the JCI as well as other accreditation programs' standards. Statistics are a component of the JCI standards found in the Quality Improvement and Patient Safety (QPS) and Management of Communication and Information (MCI) chapters of the *Joint Commission International Accreditation Standards for Hospitals, Third Edition)*. See the sidebar at the end of this chapter for more specifics.

Types of statistics

Take a look at the piles of statistical data or the studies in which your organization participates, whether for regulatory requirements or for accreditation or PI purposes. You'll see that these reports, studies, and piles of data can be neatly divided into two kinds of statistics:

- **Descriptive statistics.** This type, which is the most frequently used kind of statistics in healthcare, summarizes and organizes raw data into meaningful information. Descriptive statistics concentrates on collecting, summarizing, and displaying data. This book will focus mainly on descriptive statistics because this type is most effective for doing what you need to do: demonstrating standards compliance, measuring improvement, and providing a means of analysis.

  Examples of descriptive statistics include:
  - Patient satisfaction results
  - Mortality rates
  - Length-of-stay statistics

- **Inferential statistics.** This type of statistics emphasizes understanding an entire population based on the sample studied, or predicting future outcomes based on previous performance. In short, inferential statistics aids in decision-making based on analysis of data. Inferential statistics enables the user to make more accurate predictions or conclusions based on the data presented. These inferences are made using the mathematical concept of probability.

Two examples of inferential statistics are:

- Forecasts of next year's sales volume based on past years' sales volumes
- Predictions of election results based on sample polling data

Data: The raw material for statistics

Perhaps you're wondering, "How are statistics different from data?"

Data, at its core, is a collection of values for measurement or study. It is the raw material on which statistics are built. Without data, there is nothing for you to analyze or aggregate.

Data is composed of data points. A data point is a single specified measurement that is part of a set of data. Usually, each data point is packaged with information to help you understand it. For example, if your data comprised wait time in the emergency department (ED), a data point might be that one patient entered your ED last night, stayed for 90 minutes, and was admitted as an inpatient. Each unique bit of knowledge that you know and collect about that patient is part of that data point.

When you begin your statistical journey, be aware that:

- The data you collect should be defined. In the preceding example, before data collection began, data might be defined as total ED wait time for each patient.

- Everyone in your organization should define the same data elements in the same way. In the ED wait time example, everyone collecting data would need to be told beforehand to measure wait times from the same starting point, such as when the patient entered the ED, to the same end point, such as when the patient left the ED.

Uniform definition of data and data elements is a standards expectation of JCI and other accreditation programs. These definitions will also make life easier: If you are defining variables differently than your information management department defines them, or differently than the last group that analyzed them, then you cannot compare your results meaningfully because you will not have an apples-to-apples comparison.

All data is either **numeric** or **categorical**:

- **Numeric data**. In our example, numeric data would be wait time in minutes, patient age, admission time, and discharge time.

- **Categorical data**. Categorical data is recorded data that is not numerical—for example, whether the patient entered the ED via ambulance or was a walk-in. Similarly, the unit to which the patient was admitted would be considered categorical data because each different value could place the patient into a different category.

There are different kinds of numeric data, which are measured on different scales. The type of analysis you can perform on your data depends, in part, on what type of measurement it is. Some of these are described in the following list:

- **Nominal data**. Nominal data is assigned a number for classification purposes—for example, patient gender (i.e., 1 = female, 2 = male) or the clinic where a patient receives care (see chart).

  It does not make sense to rank nominal data because there is no hierarchy in it. As you can see in the chart, the code numbers assigned to the clinics do not measure anything; therefore, these numbers are considered nominal data.

Diagnosis-related groups are another example of data that is considered nominal.

Nominal data	
Clinic code	**Clinic name**
1	Outpatient pediatrics
2	Obstetrics
3	Main street internal medicine
4	Sport medicine clinic

- **Ordinal data**. Ordinal data indicates rank: first, second, third, and so forth. On a customer satisfaction survey, for example, ordinal data could be the numbers assigned to very satisfied (1), somewhat satisfied (2), and so on (see chart). Another example of ordinal data would be a pain scale of 1 to 10 based on the patient's perception of pain or self-reported description of pain.

Ordinal data	
Score	**Patient satisfaction level**
1	Very satisfied
2	Somewhat satisfied
3	Somewhat dissatisfied
4	Very dissatisfied

- **Interval data.** Interval data indicates a measurable unit, such as minutes, days, millimeters, liters, etc. There is no zero in interval data and no negative numbers. Examples of interval data are a patient's temperature and wait time in minutes (see chart).

Interval data	
Patient	**ED wait time (in minutes)**
A	30
B	28
C	32
D	21

- **Ratio data.** Ratio data shows a comparison and is similar to interval data in that meaningful numbers are assigned to it. However, unlike interval data, ratio data values can include zero and negative numbers. For example, profitability is considered ratio data because zero profit or negative profit is a real measurement, as the following chart shows.

Ratio data	
Fiscal year	**Cardiac center profitability**
2004	-9%
2005	0%
2006	10%
2007	12.5%

Commonly used terms

Following is a list of additional terms and concepts that you will encounter in almost every project that involves statistics. These terms also appear in later chapters of this book, so it's a good idea to get familiar with them now.

- **Aggregate:** To bring together different things into a total, mass, or whole; collected together from different sources and considered as a whole. To generate statistics, you must aggregate data.

- **Analysis:** The process of interpreting data and turning it into useful information.

- **Common cause variation:** An expected variation that occurs within all processes, which can be reduced only by changing a process.

- **Control chart:** A chart that displays variations in a process over time. Control charts are used to determine whether a variation is a normal result of a process or whether it results from special causes.

- **Mean, median, mode:** *Mean* is the average in your data set. *Median* is the middle value in a group of data. *Mode* is the most common value, or the value that occurs most frequently in your data set. Chapter 4 will explain how to use mean, median, and mode to interpret data.

- **Measurement:** In statistics, measurement is the process of recording detailed observations of the subject of interest. Measurement is not simply casual observation; it is a methodical, reproducible method of recording your observations, which forms the basis of further analysis. Medical record abstraction and direct observation of hand washing techniques are two valid methods of measurement.

- **Numerator and denominator:** In a fraction, the *numerator* is the number above the line. When calculating rates or incidents, the numerator is the number of events that is observed. The *denominator* is the number

Statistics Basics, Global Edition

below the line in a fraction and indicates the total size of a population being measured. To express the rate of hospital-acquired infection at a facility, for example, the fraction would read:

$$\frac{\text{Number of patients receiving discharge instructions}}{\text{Total number of patients discharged}}$$

Numerators and denominators are described in greater detail in Chapter 2.

- **Outlier:** A data point that is observed to be significantly farther out from the central value than the other observations in the data set. Outliers can be either higher or lower than the mean, and outliers do not indicate quality or lack thereof; they simply mark a significant aberration in the data. See Chapter 4 for more about outliers.

- **Parameter:** A parameter is a numerical measurement that describes some aspect of the population you are studying.

- **Performance measures:** When gathering healthcare PI statistics, you can report measures in two different ways:

  - *Continuous measure.* In a continuous measure, each value is a precise measurement that can fall anywhere along a continuous scale. Examples of continuous measures include wait time in minutes in the ED, and premature infant birth weight.

  - *Rate-based measure.* This is a measure of frequency. Rate-based measures identify the frequency of an event or an outcome and are expressed as ratios. A rate-based measure displays the number of events—over the entire population—that were at risk of this event or occurrence. It is displayed as a ratio—for example, falls per 1,000 patient days or cases of a do-not-use abbreviation out of a given number of discharge records.

Rate-based measures can also be described in fraction form:

$$\frac{\text{Numerator} = \text{number of occurrences}}{\text{Denominator} = \text{number of population at risk for occurrence}}$$

- **Population:** This refers to the entire group you are interested in studying. In a study of ED wait time, the population would be everyone who walked into the ED during a given survey period—for example, all of the past year.

- **Probability:** The study of chance or the likelihood of a particular outcome.

- **Ratio:** A ratio quantifies the relationship between two different counts. Ratios can be displayed as percents or as proportions.

- **Sample:** A sample is a subset of an entire population. Sampling is a widely used way of capturing data on a population when surveying the entire population would be too time-consuming or too expensive. For example, to measure compliance with the World Health Organization's guidelines for hand washing, you would need to sample because you cannot record every patient-caregiver encounter every minute of every day. Chapter 2 takes a closer look at samples and sampling.

- **Special cause variation:** A variation that results from an unexpected but explainable change in a process.

- **Standard deviation:** A measure of the variation or dispersion of data around the mean, or average value, in a data set.

    Statistics Basics, Global Edition

- **Statistical process control:** A group of statistical rules that identifies special-cause variation in data.

- **Subject:** The individual unit or event being measured. Normally, for each subject, you will collect many specific attributes. For example, if you sold six cars of different colors in one day, each of the six cars is a subject, and the description "color" is an attribute. Some of the things you collect will be numeric, such as patient age or date of admission. Other subject attributes will be descriptive, such as patient gender or primary language.

- **Variable:** In statistics, a variable is something you can measure or record about the thing you are studying or analyzing. For example, in a study of ED wait times, variables might include time of admission or day of the week.

Statistics is a process

Describing, gathering, and analyzing statistics is a process, and you and your staff must understand each step of the process.

Remember, statistics help you make informed decisions. In healthcare, your facility faces decisions every day in every department, with very little room for error. Often, these decisions are made by answering the following questions:

- Should we implement a new process?

- Will this change improve our care, our outcomes, or patient satisfaction?

The more you know about how well you're doing what you're doing, the better chance you have of moving the quality of care in the direction you want. Statistics will give you the tools to prove that care is moving in the right direction!

Let's start with an overview of a familiar improvement model (see Figure 1.1).

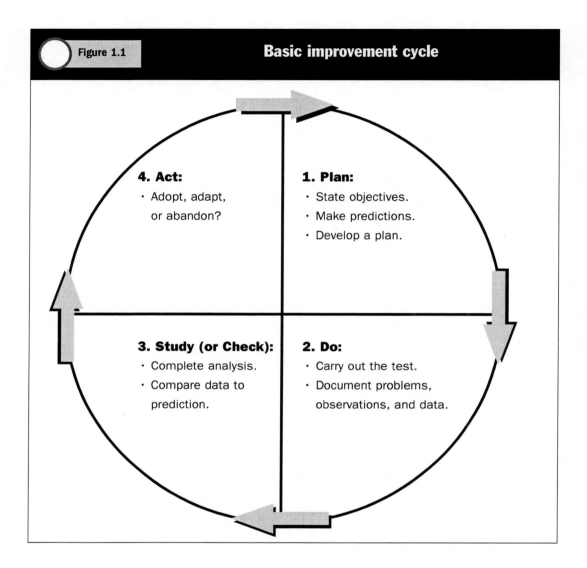

Figure 1.1   **Basic improvement cycle**

4. Act:
- Adopt, adapt, or abandon?

1. Plan:
- State objectives.
- Make predictions.
- Develop a plan.

3. Study (or Check):
- Complete analysis.
- Compare data to prediction.

2. Do:
- Carry out the test.
- Document problems, observations, and data.

If you have participated in improvement efforts in your organization, Figure 1.1 is probably very familiar to you. It may be comforting to know that the steps in a statistics cycle have a similar look and feel.

Following are the steps in the statistical process:

1. Plan your study.
2. Collect observations.
3. Code your observations as data.
4. Evaluate and analyze the data.
5. Draw conclusions and report results.

If you put statistical process steps into the improvement cycle, you'll see a good fit, as Figure 1.2 shows.

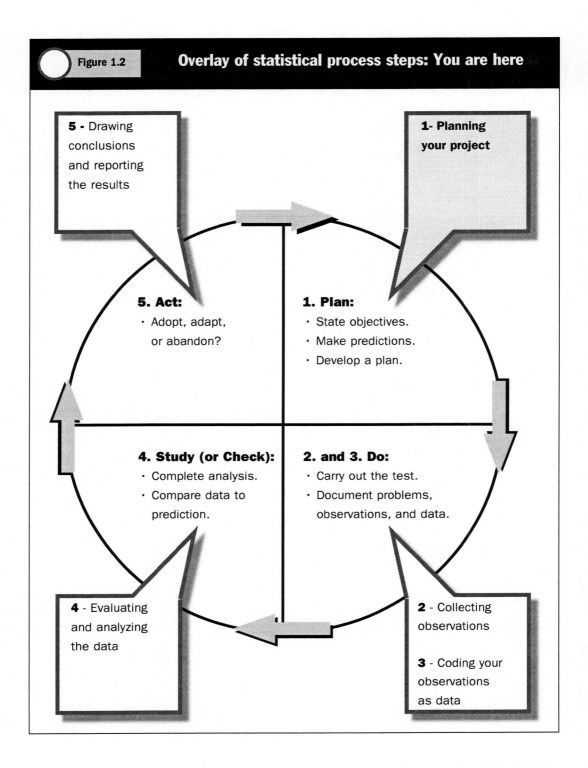

Figure 1.2 — **Overlay of statistical process steps: You are here**

5 - Drawing conclusions and reporting the results

1- Planning your project

5. Act:
- Adopt, adapt, or abandon?

1. Plan:
- State objectives.
- Make predictions.
- Develop a plan.

4. Study (or Check):
- Complete analysis.
- Compare data to prediction.

2. and 3. Do:
- Carry out the test.
- Document problems, observations, and data.

4 - Evaluating and analyzing the data

2 - Collecting observations

3 - Coding your observations as data

 Statistics Basics, Global Edition

Step 1: Plan now

The planning process generally starts when you find out that you have been appointed to manage a new measurement initiative or PI process. Perhaps your department has been asked to participate in an organizationwide PI project, and you have been tapped to manage things.

 Time spent planning now will be richly rewarded later. Although no one wants to drag out a worn-out saying, in this case it bears repeating: *If you fail to plan, plan to fail!*

Here are a few questions you will need to answer and put into your plan prior to commencing your project:

1. **What question(s) are we trying to answer?** Define your question in the form of a hypothesis or theory: Explain the effect your variables have on each other. For example, your hypothesis might be that wait time in the ED fluctuates, and that variables such as time of the day and day of the week influence the length of the wait.

2. **What is the purpose of this statistical project?** Is this a "fishing expedition" to determine the cause of a particular bad outcome or event? Or is this a controlled study to determine the effect of an improvement or new process that will be implemented in your area?

3. **How will this study be accomplished?** Is this a survey of past events or patients already seen, or is this a real-time study of patients that will be seen or treated during the duration of the project? How you plan for data collection and the timelines of your study depends heavily on the answer to this question. Before you begin, you'll need to define the steps necessary to accomplish this project.

4. **Who wants this information?** Who is your target audience: hospital administrators, staff members, external agencies, accreditation surveyors?

5. **What will the final report look like?** Will it be written or verbal? Will you give a presentation?

6. **When is the information needed?** How long is this project expected to last?

7. **What format is expected?** In other words, is there a similar study or report you could use as a template or model? Ask now before you spend time producing something your audience isn't expecting and doesn't want or need.

8. **What kind of budget or resources do you have to work with?** Who will be able to assist with the project, and how much time/other resources can you expect? Get this in writing and confirm everyone's commitment to your effort.

   In an ideal world, you will have the time and resources that are required to do a top-quality job. But in the real world of healthcare, you will in all likelihood be stretched for both time and money, yet your deadline will remain firm. The final question of this list, therefore, becomes even more important:

9. **Is there a similar study that you can use as a template?** Does another department or business partner have a similar assignment or study?

   When possible, find an external source that is already engaged in a similar study and adopt or adapt the approaches used. The value here is that someone else has done some of the design work for you—perhaps you can use the same data collection tools, the same data definitions, or the outcome measure itself.

Also, if you complete the same type of study, you may be able to use an outside organization's data as a benchmark for your results. Healthcare best practices, centers of excellence, and professional associations may be working toward common goals in similar areas. Familiarize yourself with these initiatives; invest the time and use measures or studies available in your professional community when appropriate and available. (You can find a partial listing of quality improvement agencies, data repositories, and initiatives and studies in the Appendix at the end of this book.)

When you have the answers to the questions in the preceding list, do the following:

- ☐ Put your understanding in writing.
- ☐ Put that written plan under the nose of the requester and get it signed off.

Often, things can change slightly between the time the information was requested and the time the work is completed—and you don't want to be left wondering what happened.

Also during this time, put together a timeline or generate a work plan that outlines the major steps necessary to achieve your object in the time allotted. The value of this becomes apparent when the project is rather large or new for you.

 When creating a project work plan, begin at the end. Work backward from the due date. This will help ensure that your time and resources are allotted as realistically as possible.

See Figure 1.3 for a sample work plan.

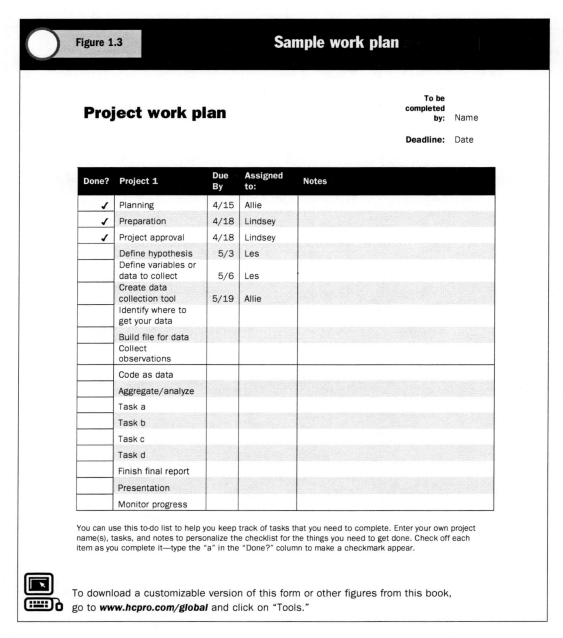

Figure 1.3 — Sample work plan

Project work plan

To be completed by: Name

Deadline: Date

Done?	Project 1	Due By	Assigned to:	Notes
✓	Planning	4/15	Allie	
✓	Preparation	4/18	Lindsey	
✓	Project approval	4/18	Lindsey	
	Define hypothesis	5/3	Les	
	Define variables or data to collect	5/6	Les	
	Create data collection tool	5/19	Allie	
	Identify where to get your data			
	Build file for data			
	Collect observations			
	Code as data			
	Aggregate/analyze			
	Task a			
	Task b			
	Task c			
	Task d			
	Finish final report			
	Presentation			
	Monitor progress			

You can use this to-do list to help you keep track of tasks that you need to complete. Enter your own project name(s), tasks, and notes to personalize the checklist for the things you need to get done. Check off each item as you complete it—type the "a" in the "Done?" column to make a checkmark appear.

To download a customizable version of this form or other figures from this book, go to **www.hcpro.com/global** and click on "Tools."

If you've got your hypothesis and variables in order, and you have planned your process for collecting useful data to generate meaningful statistics, it's time to enter the next phase of the statistics process: gathering your data. See Chapter 2.

 Statistics Basics, Global Edition

Joint Commission International expectations

Uniform definition of data and data elements is a standards expectation in the Quality and Patient Safety (QPS) chapter of the *Joint Commission International Accreditation Standards for Hospitals, Third Edition*, as shown in Figure 1.4.

It's worth expanding on QPS .4, because statistics are the backbone of this standard:[3]

You can find additional standards requirements that call for the application of statistics in the Management of Communication and Information (MCI) chapter.

Endnotes

1. Merriam-Webster's Online Dictionary © 2008, Merriam-Webster Inc., Springfield, MA. *www.m-w.com/cgi-bin/dictionary*. Accessed February 2008.
2. The Joint Commission International. *Joint Commission International Accreditation Standards for Hospitals, Third Edition*, Quality and Patient Safety chapter ©2007, Joint Commission International.
3. ibid.

Figure 1.4 | **Statistics and JCI accreditation standards**

Quality Improvement and Patient Safety (QPS) standards

Statistics are an integral part of a systemwide approach to improving patient safety. This approach includes monitoring the effectiveness of processes by collecting indicator data, analyzing this data, and implementing changes that result in improvement. QPS programs use data to identify priority issues and to demonstrate sustainable improvement.

> **QPS.4:** Individuals with appropriate experience, knowledge, and skills systematically aggregate and analyze data in the organization.
>
> **QPS.4.1:** Frequency of data analysis is appropriate to the process being studied and meets organizational requirements.
>
> **QPS.4.2:** The analysis process includes internal comparisons, comparisons with other organizations when available, and with scientific standards and desirable practices.
>
> **QPS.6:** Data is analyzed when undesirable trends and variation are evident.

Management of Communication and Information (MCI) standards

Valid statistical information—whether electronic or paper-based—is critical to effective communication throughout a hospital. Therefore, the JCI's MCI standards require that organizations must become adept at defining and capturing data, analyzing it, reporting it, and integrating it.

> **MCI.20:** Aggregate data and information support patient care, organization management, and quality management.
>
> **MCI.20.1:** The organization has a process to aggregate data and has determined what data and information will be regularly aggregated to meet the needs of clinical and managerial staff members in the organization and agencies outside the organization.
>
> **MCI.20.3:** The organization has a process for using or participating in external databases.

Source: *Joint Commission International Accreditation Standards for Hospitals, Third Edition*

 Statistics Basics, Global Edition

Data collection

What is covered in this chapter:

- Data sources

- Collecting data

- Sampling

- Building a data file

- Common risks

You've identified your project, planned it, formulated your hypothesis, gotten written approval, and created a work plan to guide your project activities and deliverables. Now it's time for the tough part: data collection. Collecting and coding data—the second and third phases of the statistical process shown in Figure 2.1—is often the most time-consuming component of the project. It can also be the most expensive. Therefore, it's important to streamline data collection as much as possible.

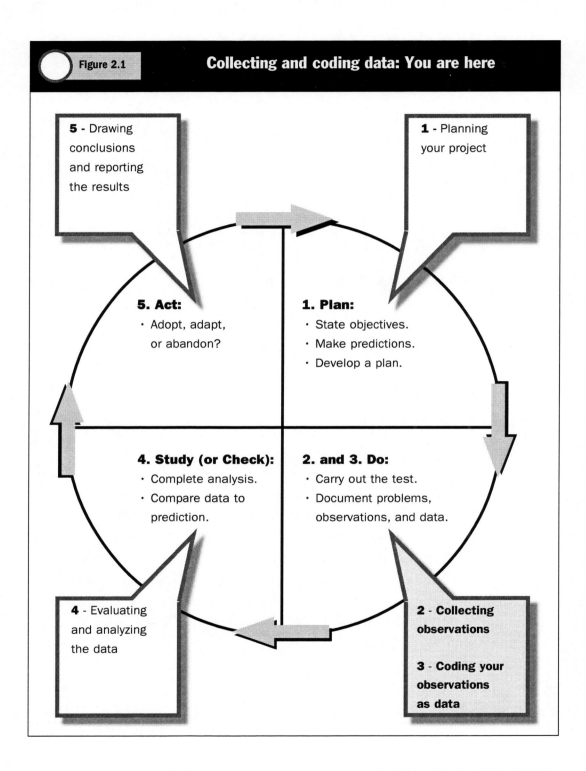

Figure 2.1

Collecting and coding data: You are here

5 - Drawing conclusions and reporting the results

1 - Planning your project

5. Act:
- Adopt, adapt, or abandon?

1. Plan:
- State objectives.
- Make predictions.
- Develop a plan.

4. Study (or Check):
- Complete analysis.
- Compare data to prediction.

2. and 3. Do:
- Carry out the test.
- Document problems, observations, and data.

4 - Evaluating and analyzing the data

2 - Collecting observations

3 - Coding your observations as data

 Statistics Basics, Global Edition

Steps in the data collection and coding phases

If you're feeling overwhelmed at the thought of simply beginning your statistics project, you can make this part of the cycle less intimidating by dividing your data collection and coding tasks into these simple steps.

1. **Identify the variables on which you are going to collect data.** What information do you need to gather? When deciding which data elements to collect, consider information that may be useful later in your project and try to include that in your up-front collection efforts.

   For example, if you're studying patient restraint usage in your hospital, for each incident in which restraint is used, you might look at the following variables:

   - Patient age
   - Gender
   - Time of day
   - Admitting physician

   This is especially important if you are collecting your data from patient records—get everything you need the first time!

2. **Create a data collection tool.** This will enable you to collect data in a consistent way. A data collection tool can be an electronic form or a paper form used by your staff to abstract medical records.

   It is important to create a data collection form that:

   - Clearly indicates what data is to be collected
   - Defines where each data piece is to come from

Your collection tool may need to include definitions of the data you are collecting. A well-designed data collection tool enables your team to gather data consistently and accurately, regardless of who is conducting the data collection.

Note: Don't skimp on this phase of the project!

Figure 2.2 shows a sample data collection form that is a simple check sheet. The person completing this type of form simply checks boxes for the variables on which data is being collected, to the extent that is feasible. For fields such as admission date and patient identifier, a blank space is available to write the requested information.

 Statistics Basics, Global Edition

Figure 2.2 **Sample check-sheet form**

ED Patient Data Collection Form

1. Patient identifier: _____

2. Date of exam _____

3. Patient gender
❑ Male   ❑ Female

4. Patient age _____ Unknown

5. Patient ethnicity/race
❑ Native American   ❑ Hispanic   ❑ African-American   ❑ Asian
❑ White (non-Hispanic)   ❑ Mixed Ethnicity/Race   ❑ Other   ❑ Unknown

6. Patient disability
❑ None   ❑ Visual   ❑ Physical   ❑ Hearing   ❑ Mental/cognitive
❑ Other   ❑ Unknown   ❑ Other Description _____

To download a customizable version of this form or other figures from this book,
go to **www.hcpro.com/global** and click on "Tools."

3. **Test your form.** After you have created your data collection form, it is vital that you test it. Testing can be simple: Ask several individuals to use the form on the same set of records. Did everyone fill out the form consistently? If not, either the form is confusing, or your data collectors have not been adequately trained.

4. **Identify your sources of data, and specify when your data was obtained.** Did you and your staff collect the information during a defined period? Was your data collected for another project? When was it collected?

    Consider multiple sources for obtaining data for your statistical analysis:

    - **Internally generated data:** This is data that can be obtained from your organization in a number of different ways.

    - **Electronic data:** Most healthcare organizations collect and store some patient-specific data on their computer systems. The advantage of capitalizing on this type of data in your collection efforts is that the data has already been collected, "cleaned," and stored in a consistent format. If you have access to reliable on-site electronic data, you can minimize your data collection expense. Armed with the data elements you wish to collect, investigate your organization's electronic medical record systems. Check your facility's billing systems, pharmacy systems, and so forth.

      Be aware that although the data is available electronically, certain expenses may be associated with accessing the data and extracting it in a format that is useful to you. If the information you need is stored in an older database, for example, you may need to enlist help from your facility's information management staff or hire someone to convert it.

 Statistics Basics, Global Edition

Make sure your electronic data actually contains the information you're looking for before committing your time and energy to gathering it.

- **Surveys:** Data is often collected from clients or patients via surveys. Patient satisfaction, for example, is often measured using forms sent to the individual's home, which are then mailed back to an external agency.

  Surveys can also be administered in writing or through personal interviews while the patient is receiving services, with the expectation that the survey form will be completed and returned prior to the patient exiting the facility. For example, you might measure clinical staff compliance with hand washing requirements by surveying patients as they exit the clinic—in other words, by asking patients, "Did you see your caregivers wash their hands before they treated you?"

 When using survey data, you must measure your response rate. The rule of thumb is that you target a response rate of 50 percent to 70 percent to ensure the data is representative of your population, and to minimize collection bias (i.e., your responses come only from a subgroup, such as very disgruntled patients, and therefore skew your data). You can improve your overall response rate by making your survey as simple as possible so respondents can complete it quickly. If it's a mailed survey, it helps to include a self-addressed stamped envelope too.

- **Manually collected data:** Manual data collection can be conducted concurrently, as care is being delivered, or retrospectively, by chart review after the fact. Either way, you need to train your data collection team members and audit their efforts to ensure that they are consistent in their approach to data collection.

- **Published data:** A number of organizations—including national health authorities in several countries—are involved in data collection and data dissemination related to healthcare outcomes. There may be opportunities to use publicly available data in your study. Several of these efforts are listed in the Appendix of this book.

  To compare your facility's performance in a particular area with organizations that are similar to yours, you will need to capture and use published data. This is referred to as benchmarking.

5. **Decide who will collect your data.** Depending on your study, data collection can be accomplished by staff members concurrently during the care process, or retrospectively, as an added step or responsibility in their day-to-day activities.

   To help ensure that staff members comply with your data collection needs and don't balk at the "extra work," make sure they're involved from the start of your project, and encourage their input. If they are involved from the start, are "owners" of the process, and understand the problem and the potential solutions, you will have greater buy-in and compliance. Audit their work regularly to ensure quality.

6. **Collect observations.** Depending on your study design, you might wish to collect data on your entire population. For example, in a small

                                    Statistics Basics, Global Edition

facility, it might be possible to collect data on every pediatric patient with asthma admitted to your emergency department or hospital.

However, the same data would be impossible to collect on every patient in a large city hospital or healthcare system. A 100 percent data collection effort is neither reasonable nor necessary for events that happen with great frequency. In circumstances such as these, you will choose to sample your data.

6a. **Sampling your data.** If you decide to sample your data, you must choose a random representative sample of sufficient size. That's easy to say, but just what is a random sample of sufficient size?

Your sample size will depend on these factors:

- The size of your population
- The level of variation within that population

There are several ways to obtain a useful sample:

- **Systematic random sampling:** Using this method, you determine the number of records in your population and divide that total by the number of records you need to sample.

  For example, if you discharged 400 patients from your hospital this quarter and you want your sample size to be 50, you divide 400 by 50 and determine that you need to select every eighth record for your sample (400 divided by 50 = 8).

  To actually select your systematic sample records, you would display your population logically—perhaps by admission date—and then pick a number between one and eight. For example, if you

picked three, you would start with the third record and select
every eighth record from there, until you'd collected data from
50 records.

- **Simple random sampling:** Using this sampling strategy, you
  select records based on a sequence provided by a random number
  generator. If you have Excel, you can use that to generate your
  sample. Several random number generators are available on the
  Internet as well.

 If you wish to use Excel to generate a random number, you will probably need to install an add-in called "Analysis ToolPak" by following
the steps below:

1. From the Tools menu, click "Data analysis."
2. If the option "data analysis" does not display, click "add-ins" and
   then on the "add-ins available" pop-up menu, click "Analysis
   ToolPak" and click "OK"
3. Highlight the medical record numbers or the records in your
   population
4. In the "tools" menu, click "data analysis"
5. Scroll down and click "random number" and follow the instructions in the wizard.

---

7. **Build a file to hold your data.** Depending on the tool you use to collect
   data, you may also need to design a file to store your data. If you have
   paper records, you will need a place to electronically enter and store
   your data for later use in the aggregation, analysis, and reporting phases
   of the project.

Regardless of where you obtain your data, you need to organize it and store it for later analysis. Your chosen vehicle for storing it could be:

- Paper logs of your observations
- Spreadsheet or database software

Storing your data electronically can expedite the next step of data collection: coding your observations.

8. **Code observations as data:** The observations you have recorded must be entered into a database or spreadsheet, such as Excel. If you are entering data manually, set up your spreadsheet using one row for each observation, and enter the variables associated with that observation across the columns (see Figure 2.3). Be sure to create headers at the top of each column and use a unique identifier for each row of data.

Figure 2.3	Sample database				
Medical record #	**Unit**	**Admit date**	**Discharge date**	**Age**	**Etc.**
347519	4 North	6/5/06	6/6/06	56	
363338	4 North	3/16/06	3/18/06	77	
299710	ICU	6/22/06	6/29/06	36	
137047	Peds	3/13/06	3/19/06	6	
333422	3 North	6/5/06	6/7/06	32	
288462	ICU	5/18/06	5/22/06	76	
419682	4 North	3/6/06	3/11/06	34	

Observations are commonly coded as numerators (such as the number of times an event was observed during the collection process) and denominators (such as the entire population observed).

Common problems in data collection

Statistics projects are performed by humans, so errors will occur. Checking your data is vital to the success of every statistics project, but this step is often overlooked and undervalued when project managers and staff members are pressed for time.

Every step in the statistics process can be prone to error. Mistakes can be introduced during observations, during the abstraction of a medical record, or in any number of other ways. Even the statistical tools you employ can and will introduce errors. You'll avoid a lot of grief if you accept this truth and check your work carefully as it progresses.

Data scrubbing

Cleaning up erroneous data, or data scrubbing, can help you avoid more errors down the line.

At some point, you have probably been in a meeting in which someone presents charts or graphs that scream trouble—perhaps the hospital's rate of falls is way up, or the length of stay is out of control, or the volume of procedures has taken an inexplicable downturn. Maybe your department has been using a stable outcome measure that suddenly goes wacky.

In this situation, the natural tendency in management oftentimes is to shoot the messenger or try to "fix" a problem without taking the time to determine whether the data that was used to prepare the analysis was correct.

If your results look amiss, eyeball the raw data. Sometimes you can easily pick out the source of your troubles—such as a patient's age recorded as 173 years old—by just scanning your raw information. Or if, for example, your facility's length of stay has risen dramatically during one month, it may be a matter of

 Statistics Basics, Global Edition

one record in which the patient's admission date was entered as the wrong year, which skewed a monthly data point.

Seemingly unrelated things might also be the cause of your negative results. If, for instance, there has been turnover among the staff charged with gathering data from medical records, the new person might not be properly trained and could be incorrectly completing data collection activities, thus skewing your outcome measure. Or perhaps a newly installed information system has inadvertently corrupted your data.

Missing data

An additional way to easily introduce errors into your process is to leave out data. Just because you got the data from your database doesn't mean there aren't problems with it. Perhaps data appears to be missing because your organization had no cases one month for the measure you are tracking. Or perhaps data was unintentionally omitted from your sample.

Validity and reliability: Two more ways to be wrong

"Is my data accurate? Can it be trusted?" Validity and reliability are the terms that address these questions:

- **Validity or accuracy:** In statistics, a valid measure is one that measures what it is supposed to measure. If you are measuring what you set out to measure, your data will have high validity.

- **Reliability or precision:** Consistency in measurement results when measuring, such as the tendency of a measurement tool to produce the same results "when it measures twice some entity or attribute believed not to have changed in the interval between measurements."[1]

  For example, a scale is unreliable if it weighs a patient three times in three minutes and gets three different weights.

Data confidentiality issues

If your statistics project involves gathering patient data, you'll need to safeguard patients' privacy. Recent cases in several countries, in which thousands or even millions of individuals' personal information was stolen, only underscore the need to protect sensitive patient information.

If you wish to use patient data internally for quality improvement purposes and other internal statistics projects, you must maintain the confidentially of the data, although you can still use the protected information in your analysis.

Don't take data confidentiality lightly. Think about ways to protect your data, your computer, and those who have access to either or both. You can safeguard that data in several ways, including the following:

- Assign each medical record number to a sequential number, and replace the medical record number with the sequential number in your file. Make sure that you, and only you, have the key.

- Make sure your project team members sign an agreement to keep sensitive data confidential.

- You can also hide or protect selected columns of sensitive information in Excel and password-protect your changes. See the following sidebar.

 Statistics Basics, Global Edition

Sidebar: Hide sensitive information

You can hide the columns that contain your patient identifiers and then protect the columns with a password. This ensures that only a person with the password can view those unique patient identifiers.

1. To hide a row or a column, click on the row (1) or column heading (2). All contents in that selected row or column will be highlighted:

Click the row (1) or column heading (2).

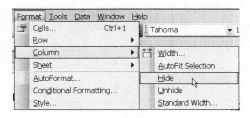

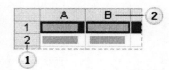

2. On the Format menu, select Row or Column, then click Hide.

3. To password-protect the selected content, do the following:

On the Tools menu, point to Protection, and then click Protect Sheet.

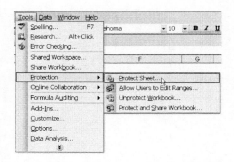

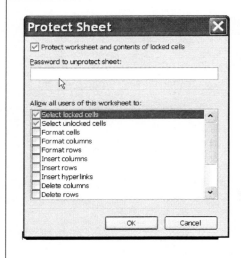

To prevent others from removing protection on that sheet, type a password, click OK, then retype the password to confirm it. Save your file. At this point, your hidden columns are protected from users who do not have your password.

An alternative way to protect numerical information, such as Social Security numbers, is to only display the last four digits of a number. This is similar to the register receipts you receive when you use a credit card for a purchase. The result of this method will display asterisks for all numbers except for the last four. To use this method, in your Excel Help pop-up, type display identification numbers and then follow the steps at the left.

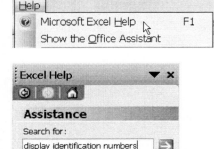

NOTE: Privacy measures vary from nation to nation, and this issue will be of increasing concern for healthcare. If you intend to obtain data from patient records, be sure to check with your legal department to determine what you must do to safeguard your data and patient information *before* starting the data collection phase of your statistics project.

Endnotes

1. Grinnell, R. M., and M. Williams (1990). *Research in Social Work: A Primer* © 1990 F.E. Peacock Itasca, IL, quoted at *http://healthlinks.washington.edu.* Web site accessed February 2008.

Data aggregation and display

What is included in this chapter:

- Summary table
- Bar chart
- Pie chart
- Histogram

- Run chart
- Scatter plot
- Control chart
- Comparison chart

For each chart, we will learn:

- What it shows
- How to create one

- When to use this chart
- When not to use it

Other thoughts for aggregation and display:

- Use the correct scale
- Comparing over time
- Comparing yourself to others (benchmarking)
- Examples of how the display affects the message

You have created your plan, created data collection tools, and collected data for a number of cases over a length of time. Now you are ready to answer the question "So what?" What does all the data mean? What is it telling you, and how will it help you make better decisions?

Data display really is where the rubber meets the road from a statistical point of view, as well as a management point of view. This chapter will show you how to turn data into information.

As Figure 3.1 shows, you are more than halfway around the statistics cycle, in the Study (or Check) phase.

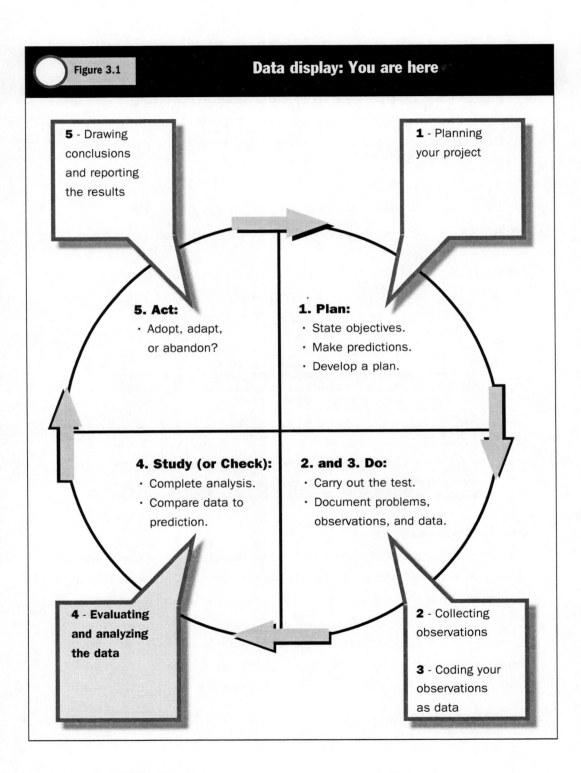

Figure 3.1

Data display: You are here

5 - Drawing conclusions and reporting the results

1 - Planning your project

5. Act:
· Adopt, adapt, or abandon?

1. Plan:
· State objectives.
· Make predictions.
· Develop a plan.

4. Study (or Check):
· Complete analysis.
· Compare data to prediction.

2. and 3. Do:
· Carry out the test.
· Document problems, observations, and data.

4 - **Evaluating and analyzing the data**

2 - Collecting observations

3 - Coding your observations as data

Chart types

Previous chapters described the value of using statistics, when statistics are necessary, the basics of data collection, sampling strategies, and how to assemble data. Chapter 3 will show you how to aggregate and display your progress in a variety of charts.

We'll start with the most basic way to aggregate and display, the summary table.

Summary table

The following is an example of a summary table. As you can see, a summary table is the most basic chart form for displaying categorical data.

Example of a summary table		
Patient satisfaction: Rating the hospital environment		
Maintaining a quiet environment	**Responses**	**%**
Never	80	6%
Sometimes	290	22%
Usually	530	40%
Always	420	32%
Responses	**1,320**	**100%**

What is a summary table?

In its simplest form, a summary table is a two-column table in which the categories to be summarized are listed in the first column, and their associated value or response is listed next to the category in the second column.

Summary tables can contain more than two columns of data—for example, patient satisfaction results can be displayed as a percentage of respondents this year compared to a percentage of respondents last year.

As shown in the preceding box, data displayed in a summary fashion gets the point across in simple terms.

When is it appropriate to use a summary table?

This chart style is most effective when used to summarize data; for example, to depict patient satisfaction surveys or patient population based on gender, payer group, native language, or other descriptors that do not lend themselves to additional statistical analysis. For example, it would not make sense to indicate that 35 percent of the patients seen in a medicine clinic are female and the remaining 65 percent are male, and that, therefore, the average patient is "mostly" male!

When is it inappropriate to use a summary table?

Although they're effective for basic displays, summary tables limit the amount and complexity of the information you can present. Readers are often left to draw their own conclusions when reviewing information in a summary table.

How do I create a summary table in Excel?

It is easy to create a summary table or any of the other chart types discussed in this chapter. Open a file in Excel on your computer, then walk through these steps using the canned charts and data provided, or use your own data. Either way, you will be surprised at how quickly you can generate effective charts.

Creating a summary table is similar to entering data. If your data has already been summarized, simply enter your data and format your cells to display in text, date, or numeric format. When preparing any chart, remember to label it, as well as the column headings and any other aspect of the data that would not be obvious if an uninformed user were to read it.

TIP Ideally, a chart should be able to stand alone and need no further explanation from the presenter.

If your data is more complex, you may need to summarize it prior to preparing your summary table. Thankfully, spreadsheet packages, such as Excel, make this very easy and quick for you.

Summarizing the contents of a row of data using a formula

This is actually easier than it sounds. And summarizing contents makes it easy to do common things such as adding or averaging the data in your spreadsheet. Follow the steps in Figure 3.2 to summarize the contents of a row of data using a formula.

Bonus Excel tip: How to calculate average, minimum, maximum, or count

You can use the steps outlined in Figure 3.2 to perform four other common calculations:

- **Average:** Calculates the average of the selected range of cells.

- **Count:** Counts the number of numeric values in the selected range of cells. Non-numeric or blank cells are not counted.

- **Maximum:** Identifies the maximum value in the selected range of cells.

- **Minimum:** Finds the minimum value in the selected range of cells.

To perform one of these functions, use the steps outlined in Figure 3.2, but instead of clicking the Auto Sum button, click the down arrow to the right of it. You will see the following drop-down menu:

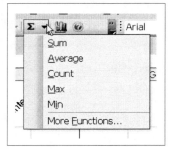

Click on the function you want and press Enter. The math is done for you.

    Statistics Basics, Global Edition

 Figure 3.2 **Summarizing data using a formula**

To summarize your data using a formula, follow these steps:

1. Enter your data in rows and columns.

	A	B	C	D	E	F
1						
2						
3	Volunteer Hours Worked Per Week					
4		Volunteer A	Volunteer B	Volunteer D	Volunteer D	
5	January					
6	Week 1	8	4	16	4	
7	Week 2	8	0	8	4	
8	Week 3	8	4	4	4	
9	Week 4	8	4	4	2	
10						

2.

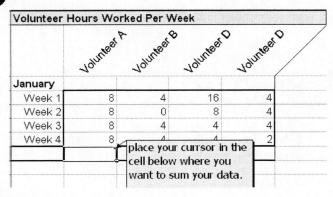

Volunteer Hours Worked Per Week

	Volunteer A	Volunteer B	Volunteer D	Volunteer D
January				
Week 1	8	4	16	4
Week 2	8	0	8	4
Week 3	8	4	4	4
Week 4	8	4	4	2

place your cursor in the cell below where you want to sum your data.

3. Click the AutoSum button.

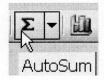

AutoSum

Excel will outline the range of edits to sum. You can modify this range if necessary.

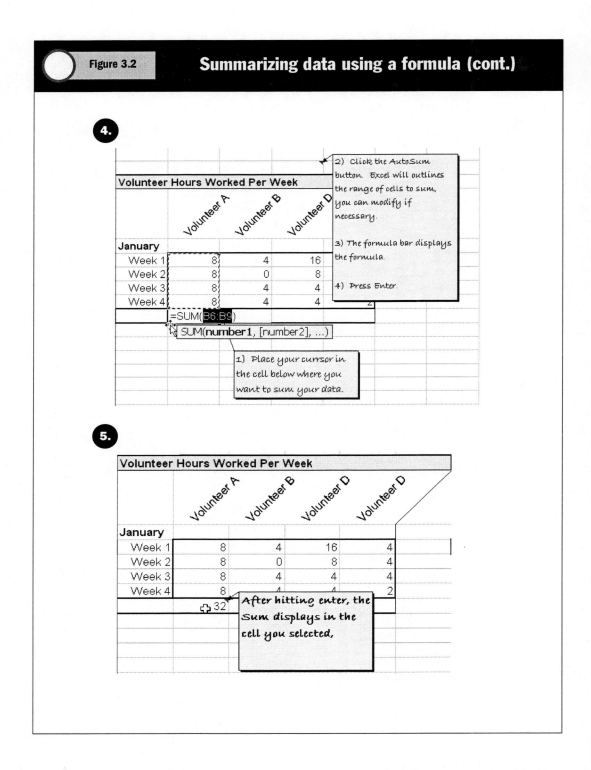

Figure 3.2 — Summarizing data using a formula (cont.)

4.

Volunteer Hours Worked Per Week

2) Click the AutoSum button. Excel will outlines the range of cells to sum, you can modify if necessary.

3) The formula bar displays the formula.

4) Press Enter.

	Volunteer A	Volunteer B	Volunteer D
January			
Week 1	8	4	16
Week 2	8	0	8
Week 3	8	4	4
Week 4	8	4	4

=SUM(B6:B9)

SUM(**number1**, [number2], …)

1) Place your cursor in the cell below where you want to sum your data.

5.

Volunteer Hours Worked Per Week

	Volunteer A	Volunteer B	Volunteer D	Volunteer D
January				
Week 1	8	4	16	4
Week 2	8	0	8	4
Week 3	8	4	4	4
Week 4	8	4	4	2
	32			

After hitting enter, the Sum displays in the cell you selected,

Statistics Basics, Global Edition

Line graph (also called a run chart)

A line graph, or run chart, is another simple, effective way of displaying data. Line graphs are also sometimes referred to as trend line charts. The following is an example of a line graph.

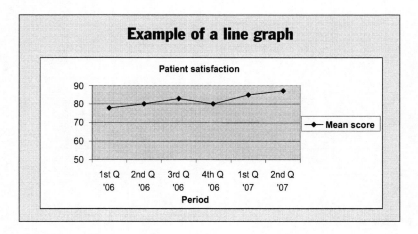

What is a line graph?

Line graphs are a good way to show data variation over time. When creating a line graph, you can get your first look at your data, portrayed as a picture, and begin to see what your data is telling you.

When is it appropriate to use a line graph?

Several types of line graphs are useful in different situations:

- **Single-line graph:** This will show how a single variable changes across the horizontal axis (x-axis). Single-line graphs are often used to show improvement or variation over time.

- **Multiple-line graph:** This type of graph allows you to show the performance of multiple variables over time, or over the horizontal axis (x-axis). Following is an example of a multiple-line graph.

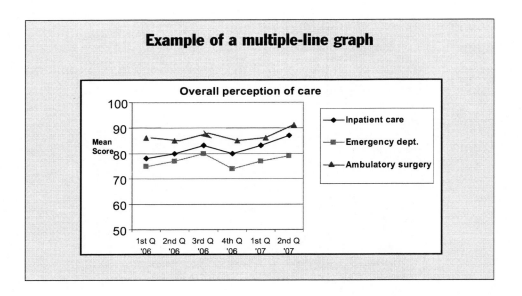

Area graph

Conceptually the same as the single- or multiple-line graph, an area graph is used to visually emphasize your point. For example, if you are comparing your department to an external benchmark, and you have demonstrated significant progress on that effort, an area graph will tell your story more emphatically than would a line graph alone.

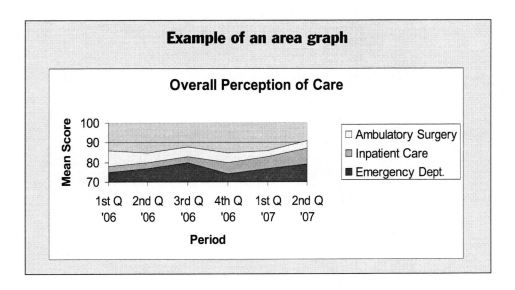

Note: Do not use an area graph if your lines cross one another. In an area graph, the space, or area, between the lines is important. You can visually emphasize that area in an area graph as opposed to the simpler multiple-line graph.

Control chart

A control chart is a line graph that shows where statistical analysis has been performed on data to identify a variation in the process and to distinguish whether that variation is due to common causes or special circumstances. A control chart is a graphical display of process stability or instability over time. You create a control chart by starting with a run chart. You can create a simple one using Excel. (The concept of statistical process control will be further described in Chapter 4.)

The following is an example of a control chart.

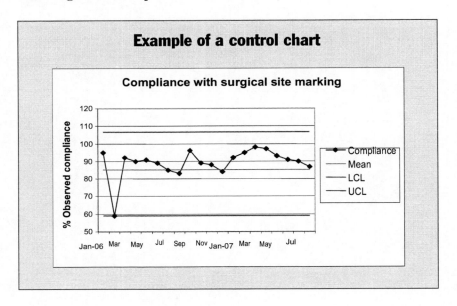

Example of a control chart

When is it inappropriate to use a control chart?

This chart type is easy to create and is familiar to most people, but it can become confusing or "noisy" if you attempt to display too many variables on one graph. Lines become tangled and no visual conclusions can be drawn.

In addition, although software such as Excel will allow you to soup up your graphical presentations by easily creating 3-D graphs, sometimes you must resist the temptation. Fancy charts may look great in an overhead presentation, but they can be difficult to interpret. And you don't want your audience to spend valuable presentation time trying to grasp simple things such as direction and scale, instead of focusing on the message your data conveys.

How do I create a control chart in Excel?

See Figure 3.3 for a step-by-step guide to creating line graphs and control charts that will not cause audience confusion.

 Statistics Basics, Global Edition

Figure 3.3

Creating a line graph

To create a line graph in Excel, follow these steps:

1. Open the Excel spreadsheet that contains the data you want to use for a line graph.

2. Make sure your spreadsheet data is formatted so that there are data labels directly next to each row and column of data. Excel will automatically create legends and label your axis on your graph if you label each column and row appropriately. No blank rows or columns should separate your data from its appropriate description or label.

Month	Inpatient Falls/1,000 days	Benchmark
Jan	4	3.4
Feb	7	3.4
Mar	2	3.4
April	6	3.4
May	3	3.4
June	4	3.4
July	4	3.4
Aug	3	3.4
Sept	2	3.4
Oct	3	3.4
Nov	2	3.4
Dec	3	3.4

3. Using your cursor, highlight the data you want to chart and the row and column labels for that data, as shown in the preceding figure. Select the Chart Wizard option from your toolbar.

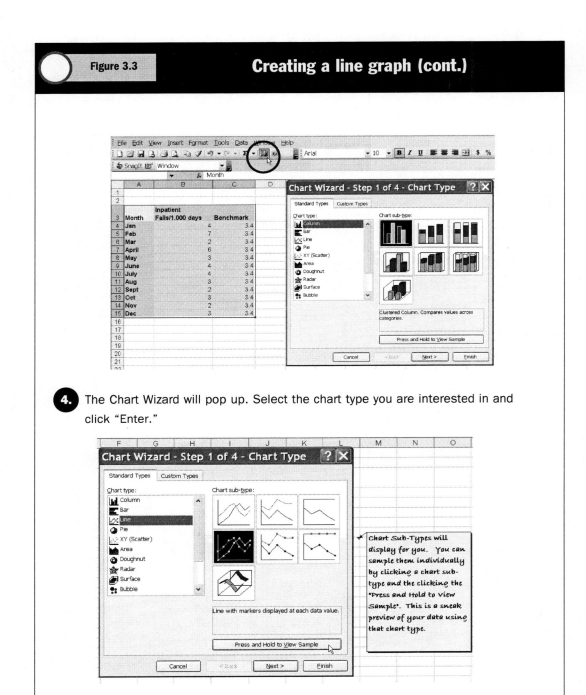

Figure 3.3 — Creating a line graph (cont.)

4. The Chart Wizard will pop up. Select the chart type you are interested in and click "Enter."

Chart Sub-Types will display for you. You can sample them individually by clicking a chart sub-type and the clicking the "Press and Hold to View Sample". This is a sneak preview of your data using that chart type.

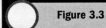 **Figure 3.3**

Creating a line graph (cont.)

5. You can sample the chart sub-
types individually by clicking a
chart subtype and then clicking the
"Press and Hold to View Sample"
button. You'll see a sneak preview
of your data using that chart type.

6. Click "Next" to create your chart.

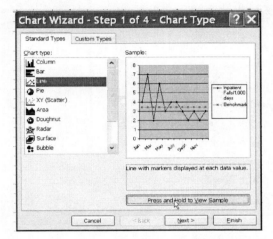

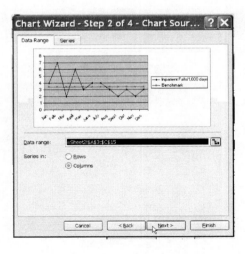

7. The Chart Wizard will lead
you through three more
screens that will allow you to
add things such as titles and
axis labels. Click "Next" to
continue after supplying the
requested information.

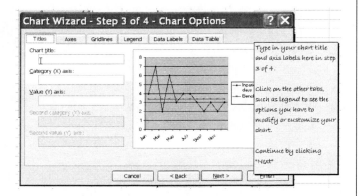

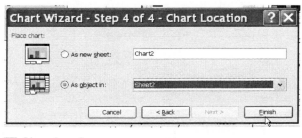

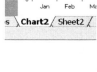

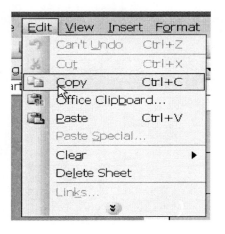

Figure 3.3 — **Creating a line graph (cont.)**

8. At this point, you are asked where you want your chart created. You have two options. You can create it right in the sheet you are working in by clicking the button labeled "As object in," or you can create the chart in a brand-new worksheet by clicking the button labeled "As new sheet." The new worksheet will be in the same file in which you are currently working, and you will see the chart as a new tab in your existing file.

9. When your chart has been created, you can copy and paste it into a Word or PowerPoint document by clicking on the outside edge of your chart and then using the Edit–Copy and Edit–Paste buttons on your toolbar.

©2008 HCPro, Inc. **Statistics Basics, Global Edition**

Pie chart

Following is an example of a pie chart.

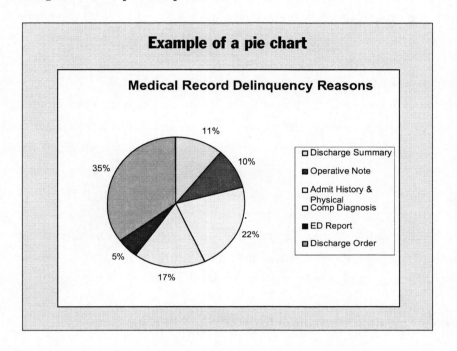

Example of a pie chart

Medical Record Delinquency Reasons

- □ Discharge Summary
- ■ Operative Note
- □ Admit History & Physical
- □ Comp Diagnosis
- ■ ED Report
- ▨ Discharge Order

What is a pie chart?

A pie chart is a very effective way to display the various parts that make up a whole. It's also a clear way to show proportions. For example, if you have collected data on your delinquent medical records and have tabulated the missing elements of each medical record, you can use a pie chart to display the proportion of each missing element.

When is it appropriate to use a pie chart?

Use a pie chart when you want to display the parts that make up a single variable. If you have multiple variables, such as a payer mix for your different clinics or reasons for medical record delinquencies, you can display several pie charts on one page. This allows the reader to compare the differences between them visually.

It almost goes without saying, but the parts you are displaying in your pies must total 100 percent of the variable you are describing. No partial pies! Also, don't forget to label the pieces of the pie. You can label the pie pieces in the legend, or, if using Excel, you can label each piece as you go.

When is it inappropriate to use a pie chart?

The variable you are measuring cannot be divided into too many subgroups, or the difference between the pieces of the pie becomes blurred. There is a way around this, though. Say, for example, that in the patient mix for your hospital, you have five major patient types that make up 90 percent of the population you serve, but there are also an additional dozen patient types that are reported very infrequently. You might group these last 12 patients under one heading called "other" or "additional patient types," and then simply footnote the patients represented in that grouping somewhere in your presentation. Don't let the minority detract from the message of the majority.

How do I create a pie chart in Excel?

To create a pie chart in Excel, follow these steps:

1. Open the Excel file containing the data you want to graph.

2. Highlight the data you want to chart. Include the labels for the rows and columns in the area you highlight.

3. Click the Chart Wizard in your toolbar and select the pie chart.

4. Complete steps 2 through 4 of the wizard, modifying or adding information as desired. Click "Next" and then "Finish" when you are on step 4 of the wizard.

5. To impress your colleagues, or to emphasize a particular section of the pie chart for your audience, you can "pull out" one slice of the pie, as shown on the next page, by first clicking on the pie and then clicking on the specific slice of the pie you want to highlight, and dragging and dropping it away from the rest of the pie.

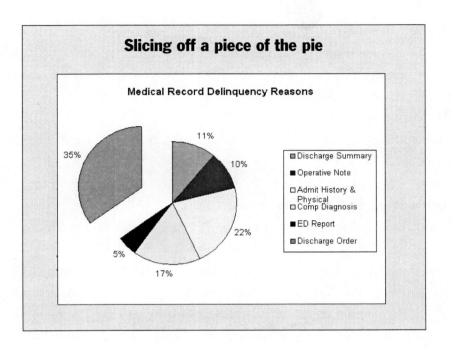

Bar chart

Below is an example of a bar chart.

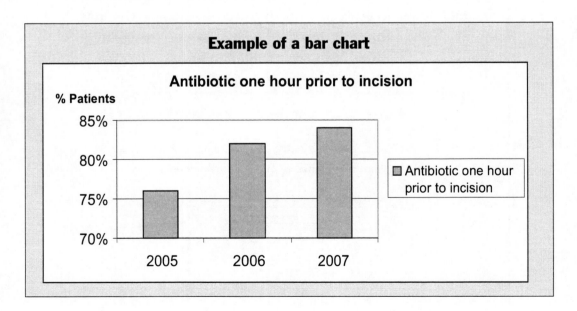

What is a bar chart?

Bar charts come in many shapes, sizes, and styles. At their most basic, they display one bar for each value of the variable in your data set. Bar charts are an effective way to display categorical data.

In a bar chart, columns are separated from each other by a small amount of space.

When is it appropriate to use a bar chart?

There are many subtypes of bar charts, each useful in different applications:

- **Vertical bar chart:** This is arguably the most common form of bar chart. In the vertical bar chart shown, the reader easily sees the taller bars as significant or different from the others in the group. In our culture, taller is bigger, and visually, it makes more of an impact. (The chart on the preceding page is an example of a vertical bar chart.)

- **Horizontal bar chart**: The same information can be displayed horizontally as well as vertically. You should consider using a horizontal bar chart if the length of the bar signifies something such as time, as shown in the following chart.

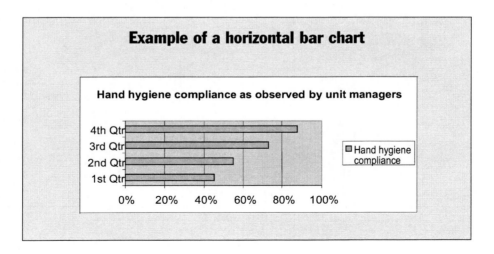

                       Statistics Basics, Global Edition

- **Stacked bar chart:** In a stacked bar chart, sometimes called a segmented bar chart, each variable, or bar, on the chart is subdivided using different colors or shadings to describe the unique cases, or attributes, that comprise each variable, as shown here:

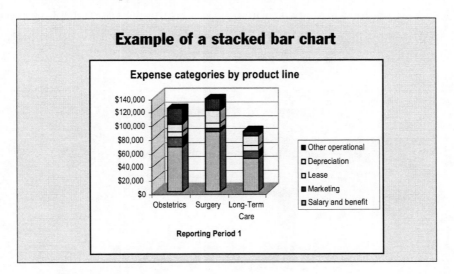

Example of a stacked bar chart

Expense categories by product line

Reporting Period 1

Legend:
- Other operational
- Depreciation
- Lease
- Marketing
- Salary and benefit

- **Multiple bar chart:** This is an effective way to group more complex data for display purposes. In a multiple bar chart, data must be divided into subgroups. Clear and proper labeling is critical to the effectiveness of a multiple bar chart, as shown in the following chart.

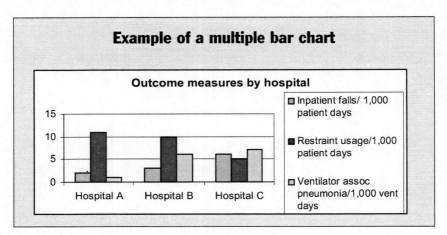

Example of a multiple bar chart

Outcome measures by hospital

Legend:
- Inpatient falls/ 1,000 patient days
- Restraint usage/1,000 patient days
- Ventilator assoc pneumonia/1,000 vent days

- **Pareto diagram:** A Pareto diagram is a specialized type of bar chart that displays nominal data. The bars in the chart do not convey order or importance (as compared to a bar chart in which the horizontal axis represents time). Pareto diagrams may be used for results of a survey on color choice for a new automobile, for example. When displaying data in a Pareto chart, you normally order your data from lowest to highest so that the chart conveys order from least to greatest, as shown:

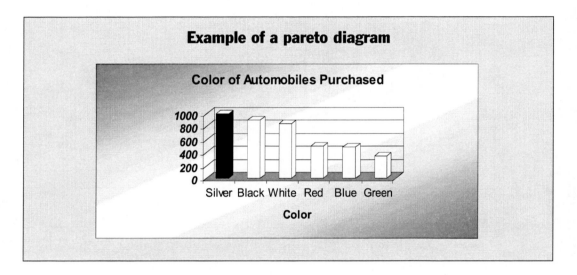

How do I create a bar chart in Excel?

Follow the instructions for creating a line graph, but use the toolbar to select one of the bar chart styles from the Chart Wizard. At this point, you can further customize the bar chart until you are satisfied, as explained in Figure 3.4.

Data aggregation and display

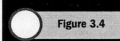 **Customizing a bar chart**

Once you have created your bar chart using steps 1 through 4 of the Chart Wizard, you can modify the look of things to suit your preferences. Changing charts of all types is easy. For example, to change the color scheme used in the chart you have created, simply click on the bar you want to change. If you click any bar once, you should see all bars in that series highlighted or selected, and you will know you selected all bars if they have dots, as shown below.

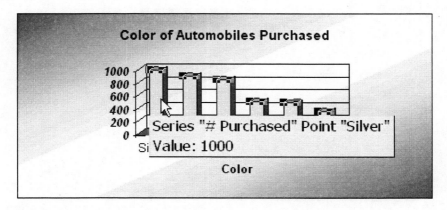

Once your bars are highlighted, click "Format" in the toolbar and then click "Selected Data Series."

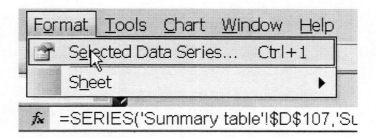

In the window that pops up, you will see your chart. Select the tab at the top, labeled "Patterns," and select a new color—red, for example. Click "OK" and all your bars should be red.

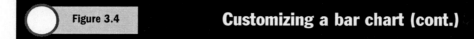

Figure 3.4 — Customizing a bar chart (cont.)

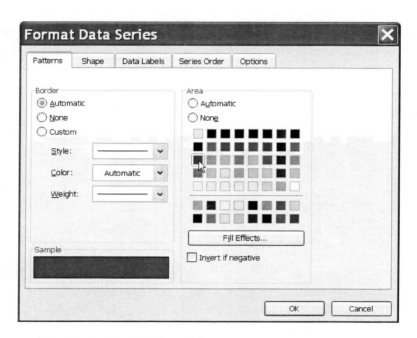

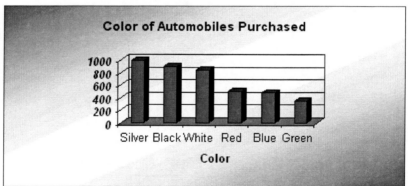

You can use the same method to change anything you see on your graph. You first select the item you want to modify, click "Format," and then check out your options on each tab of the pop-up window.

 Statistics Basics, Global Edition

Histogram

Following is an example of a histogram.

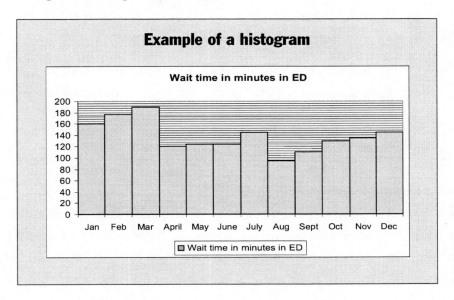

What is a histogram?

A histogram is really a subtype of the bar chart. Histograms are used to demonstrate frequency distribution of numerical data or variables.

In a histogram, there is usually no space separating the columns in the graph.

When is it appropriate to use a histogram?

Histograms are often used to display frequency, or changes in the data that occur over a time. Time periods are displayed over the horizontal axis (x axis).

When is it inappropriate to use it?

Scale is important in a histogram. Your readers will form conclusions about the data you are presenting based on the visual effect the histogram makes.

Differences in outcome measures can be accentuated (or exaggerated) based on the scale you choose.

- For small data sets, use a small number of intervals

- For large data sets, use more intervals, round numbers, and groupings of variables that are large enough to convey the differences in the data

- Remember to label both the horizontal and vertical axes, as well as the variables displayed

How do I create a histogram in Excel?

There is no chart type labeled "histogram" in Excel. To create a histogram, select one of the available bar chart formats and create a chart. Once your chart is created, eliminate the blank spaces between the columns by clicking on one of the bars in your chart and then selecting "Format" and "Selected Data Series" from the menu at the top of your screen, as shown here:

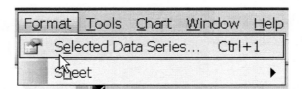

Once you see the pop-up with your chart, click on the tab labeled "Options." In that window, change the "Gap Width" to zero as shown:

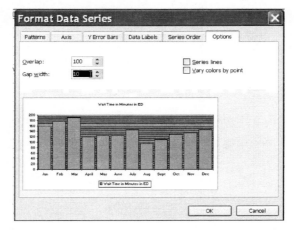

©2008 HCPro, Inc. **Statistics Basics, Global Edition**

Scatter plot

Here is an example of a scatter plot.

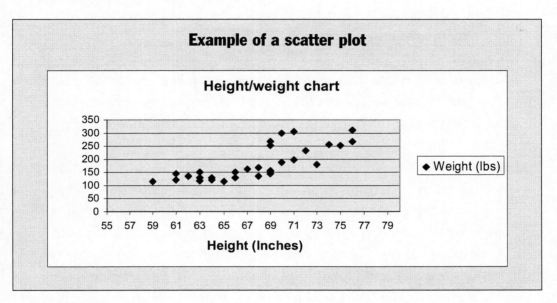

What is a scatter plot?

A scatter plot (sometimes called an XY chart) allows you to quickly analyze the correlation between two or more data series. It allows you to see trends or associations between different numeric variables, such as interval or ratio data.

When is it appropriate to use a scatter plot?

A scatter plot shows how results or outcomes on one numeric variable relate to a different numeric variable. It can display possible correlations between your two variables.

In addition to displaying a possible correlation in your data, scatter plots also can show the frequency of reported results. If you look at the height/weight sample shown, you can see that most patients' height falls somewhere between really tall and really short, so most observations are grouped in the middle.

To determine whether there is a statistical correlation between the two variables presented, you must go a step further and plot a regression line on the data. Again, Excel can automatically create a linear regression line (also called a trend line) on your data.

A linear regression line when plotted on your scatter plot can slope either up to the right, in which case it is called a **positive correlation,** or down to the right, in which case you can say you have a **negative correlation** of the data.

Linear regression is a technique of fitting the best possible straight line through a series of points. Linear regression is based on the assumption that only one of the variables can be normally distributed; the other variable must be "fixed" experimentally. Both weight and length are normally distributed in the example, however. Therefore, for height and weight, we may choose to use a statistical tool called logarithmic regression. This is a specialized trend line that creates a best-fit curved line that illustrates the relationship between data values.

When is it inappropriate to use a scatter plot?

Scatter plots cannot display categorical data in meaningful ways. If you chart your data using a scatter plot, and the result looks something like rain on a car windshield or a circular clump of data points on a chart, perhaps there is no correlation in the two reported variables, and a more effective display of the data may be in order.

How do I create a scatter plot in Excel?

Follow these steps to create a scatter plot in Excel:

1. Open the Excel file containing the data you want to graph.

2. Highlight the data you want to chart, including the data labels for the rows and columns in the area you highlight.

3. Click the Chart Wizard in your toolbar and select the "XY Scatter" chart type.

4. Complete steps 2 through 4 of the wizard, modifying or adding information as desired. Click "Next" and then "Finish" when you are on step 4 of the wizard.

5. Using Excel, you can add a trend line to your scatter plot by following these steps:

    5a. Click on the scatter plot in which you want to add the trend line.

    5b. In the top menu bar, click "Chart" and "Add Trend-line". The "Add Trend-line" pop-up dialog box will appear. Several trend-line options are available in Excel.

For a scatter plot, you may want to choose "Linear." A linear trend line creates a best-fit straight line that displays how values in your data set either increase or decrease at a steady pace, as shown here:

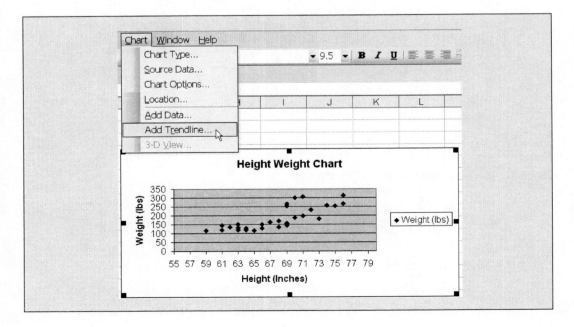

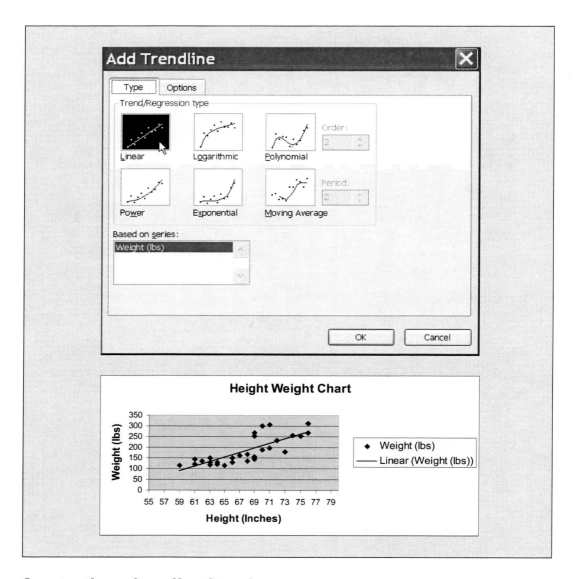

Suggestions for effective charts

Following are some tips for charting your data in the most effective way:

- **Make sure each chart can stand alone.** Your goal is simplicity. If a colleague picked up a copy of the chart and reviewed it, could he or she understand it without explanation? Remember that some members of your audience will cease listening to you, when presented with information such as a colorful chart, and will instead start to review your printed material. So the material must be able to speak for itself. Make sure labels, titles, dates, and project information are displayed on the chart correctly.

- **Include a date on the page displaying the chart.** That way, if you update your data and revise your reports, you can easily communicate which copy is the most recent.

- **Insert the path and file name in each chart you prepare.** Think of this as insurance for preventing rework later. Including the path and file name is a simple way to avoid having to re-create a chart from scratch six months from now, when you need to update data and can't remember where you stored your chart or what it was named.

- **Use the templates in this book.** If you are asked to create a chart to display the results of the project data you are working on, do the following:

  1. Look through the examples of charts in this chapter.

  2. Select the one that is most appropriate to the data you are presenting.

  3. Follow the creation instructions, then save.

  4. Replace the data labels in the example with your own material and then key in your data, expanding the range as necessary to include all of your data.

If work has been done on this project by someone whose information was clear and well accepted by your audience, consider using his or her files as a template.

If you are under pressure to get your charts done quickly, it is easy to miss obvious errors. Prior to presenting your material, take a critical look at it. Does it make sense? If there are data-entry errors or other glaring mistakes, make sure *you* find them first! When possible, have someone else look at your work, including the raw data table. It is often easier for others to find mistakes.

If you are presenting multiple analyses or multiple charts and graphs, remember the acronym "KIS," for "Keep It Simple." Keep fonts, colors, and styles consistent. That way, you won't accidentally shift your audience's attention away from what you are trying to say with your presentation.

Checklist of things to include in your report

The following is a checklist that you might find handy when creating your report:

❑ The title should be clear. Include whether the data is a sample or the entire measurable data set.

❑ Label the primary axis and secondary axis, and if the scale is a unit of measure, such as temperature, make sure the unit is displayed.

❑ Make sure the descriptions in the legend are meaningful. Excel can create them automatically for many chart types.

Other tips for aggregation and display

Here are some additional aggregation and display tips that you may find helpful:

• **Use the correct scale.** Size counts, as the two graphs in Figure 3.5 show. Both use the same data, but one appears to show a process with little variation, and the other shows a process that is in decline. The difference between the two charts is simply the scale that was chosen to use for display—starting the display at a point above zero can allow the same data to show greater detail.

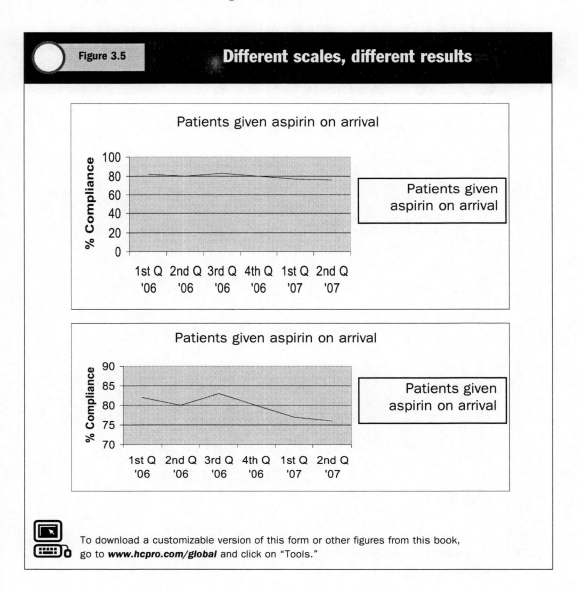

Figure 3.5 **Different scales, different results**

- **Compare your performance over time.** When comparing yourself over time, use enough data to show trends. Again, the tools and techniques you use to display your data will affect the message they send. In the example in Figure 3.6, a limited view of the available historical data skews the message.

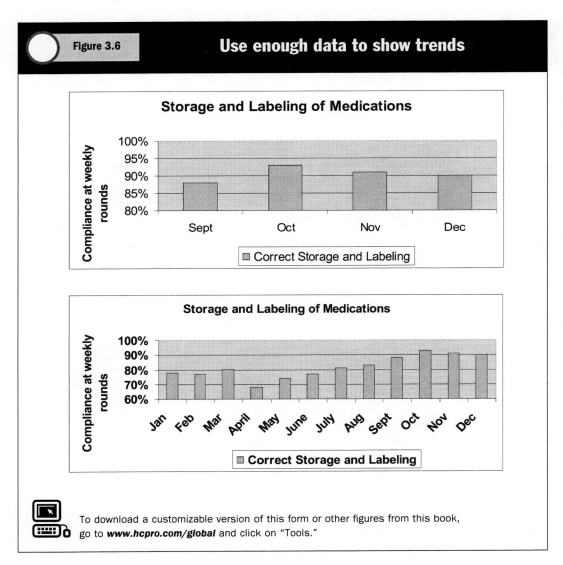

Figure 3.6 — **Use enough data to show trends**

To download a customizable version of this form or other figures from this book, go to **www.hcpro.com/global** and click on "Tools."

 Statistics Basics, Global Edition

- **Internal comparisons.** A powerful and often underused technique to elicit changes in behavior is a visual comparison of yourself to your hospital's performance. In Figure 3.7, the restraint data, which is collected by hospital, is displayed for each hospital over time. Differences between hospitals become apparent.

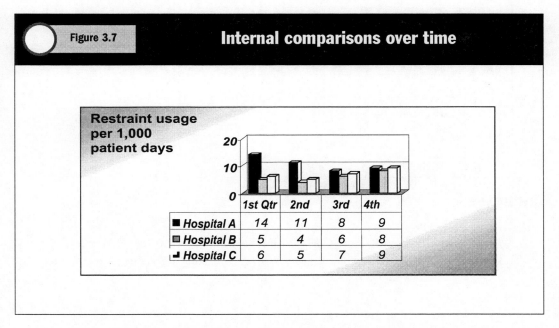

Figure 3.7	Internal comparisons over time

Restraint usage per 1,000 patient days

	1st Qtr	2nd	3rd	4th
■ Hospital A	14	11	8	9
▨ Hospital B	5	4	6	8
◢ Hospital C	6	5	7	9

- **Compare yourself to others (benchmarking).** Benchmarking, or comparing your performance to that of a relevant group, is both good business and a requirement of the Joint Commission standards. Benchmarking can be displayed in a number of chart formats. Figure 3.8 shows how a multiple-line graph can be used to display organizational performance against benchmark data.

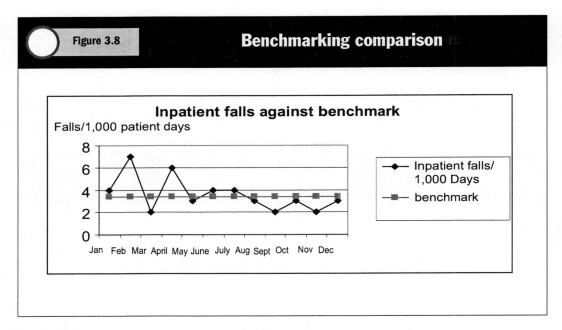

Figure 3.8 **Benchmarking comparison**

Inpatient falls against benchmark
Falls/1,000 patient days

Endnotes

1. *Benchmarking Basics, A Resource Guide for Healthcare Managers*, by Cynthia Barnard,
© 2006 HCPro, Inc., takes an in-depth look at benchmarking in the healthcare industry.

Data analysis

What is included in this chapter:

- Central tendency

  - Mean   - Mode
  - Median   - Rank and percentile

- Variation—how to measure

  - Range   - Standard deviation

For each we will learn:

- What it is

- How you can use this to interpret your performance

- When it is appropriate to use this statistical tool

- How to do it

- Statistical Process Control—rules for determining special cause variation

- Taking it to the next level—where to find additional resources when more complex statistical correlation methods are necessary

---

Analysis is the phase that follows data aggregation and display, and Chapter 4 is the what-do-you-do-next chapter.

This chapter explores common statistical measures, including mean, median, and mode, range, percentile, variance, and standard deviation. This stuff is meaningful and somewhat scary for non-numbers-type people. Don't be frightened: Remember, this book is meant to be an introduction to statistics and is geared to the average user.

Much of what you'll learn in this chapter meets the 80/20 rule: You will learn about the tools you will use for improvement efforts 80 percent of the time. Chapter 4 will touch on the 20 percent stuff—which you will seldom (if ever) be called upon to use—but won't go into these concepts in depth. The additional resources listed in the Appendix can point you toward the next level of statistical analysis.

What does data analysis mean, and what do you need to know?

As Figure 4.1 shows, you are still in the evaluating-and-analyzing-the-data phase of the process, the phase associated with the Study (or Check) phase of the cycle.

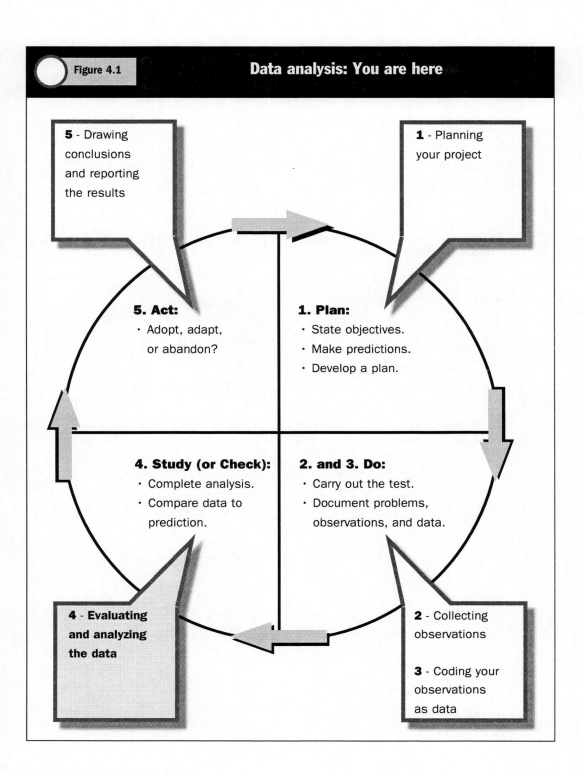

Figure 4.1

Data analysis: You are here

5 - Drawing conclusions and reporting the results

1 - Planning your project

5. Act:
- Adopt, adapt, or abandon?

1. Plan:
- State objectives.
- Make predictions.
- Develop a plan.

4. Study (or Check):
- Complete analysis.
- Compare data to prediction.

2. and 3. Do:
- Carry out the test.
- Document problems, observations, and data.

4 - Evaluating and analyzing the data

2 - Collecting observations

3 - Coding your observations as data

How do you determine whether what you are seeing in the display of your data is a real problem, statistically speaking? This chapter, in a nutshell, will show you how to use analytical tools—statistical tools—to determine whether your data demonstrates a problem that is statistically significant.

To perform statistical calculations in Excel, you must first enable or install the Analysis Toolpak. This free add-in is available when you install Microsoft Excel. To add the Analysis Toolpak, follow these steps:

1. In the Tools menu, click "Add-Ins."

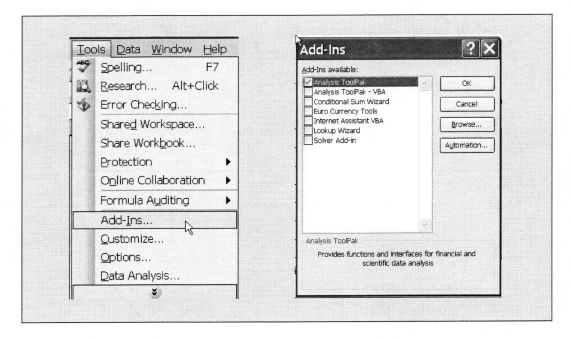

2. In the "Add-Ins available" pop-up box, check the "Analysis Toolpak" checkbox, and then click "OK." You may need to click "Browse" to locate it.

3. If you see a message that tells you the Analysis Toolpak is not currently installed on your computer, click "Yes" to install it.

 Statistics Basics, Global Edition

4. After completing these steps, you should see "Data Analysis" as an option at the bottom of the Tools menu. We will be using the data analysis tools for the examples in this chapter.

Now it's time to dig into **descriptive** and **inferential** statistics, which were defined in Chapter 1. Descriptive statistics summarize and organize raw data into meaningful information, describing the general features of the data and of the data distribution. Inferential statistics describe the strength of a relationship in the data.

Let's start with some basic descriptive statistics. These statistics are commonly used and can be quickly calculated using.the analysis tools in Excel.

Measures of central tendency

Statistical tools can be grouped based on what they are fundamentally trying to accomplish. Measures of central tendency are statistical methods that help measure the properties of your observations or data points. Most business data, as well as much of the data you will be working with, will tend to center on a particular number or value.

There are several measures of central tendency.

Mean
What is the mean?
The mean represents the average value in a data set.

When is it appropriate to use the mean?
This is a very frequently used statistic in healthcare and elsewhere. Mean measurements, such as the average wait time in the emergency department or the average length of stay (LOS) on an inpatient care unit, are no doubt familiar to you.

Mean is familiar to all, easy to calculate and understand, and therefore used more frequently than all other measures of central tendency. Your mean can determine whether additional action is needed to improve performance in the given area, or whether current measures are adequate.

However, it is important to understand that the mean can be distorted significantly if you have even a couple of erroneous data observations in your set. For example, the average LOS for a unit can swing wildly if the wrong year is recorded for one patient stay.

When is it inappropriate to use the mean?

The mean is meaningless when your data is nominal. For example, it would be pointless to calculate the average outpatient clinic name.

How do you calculate the mean?

To manually calculate the mean, add your individual data points and divide that sum by the number of observations. To calculate a mean in Excel, follow these steps:

1. Place your cursor in the cell directly below the column of data you wish to average (if you are averaging a column, or if you are averaging the values in a row of data, place your cursor in the blank cell to the right of your last data value).

2. Click on the down arrow to the right of the Sum button in your toolbar and then click on "Average" in the drop-down menu.

3. Click "Enter."

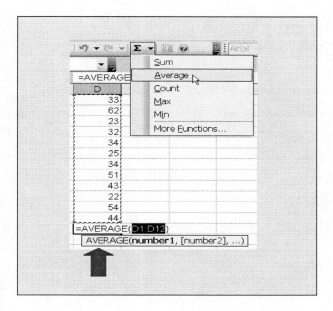

Median

What is the median?

The middle value in a group of data is the median value.

When is it appropriate to use the median?

As a measure of central tendency, the median is useful when your data contains extreme values at either the high or the low end. When calculating the median value of a data set, you eliminate the bias introduced by data errors or extreme values in the data. In the average LOS example used earlier, you could use the middle value to eliminate the bias introduced by the record that erroneously reported a LOS of more than a year.

The median is usually the best measure of central tendency when used with ordinal data, such as results of a customer satisfaction survey (satisfied, very satisfied, etc.).

When is it inappropriate to use the median?

It's important to remember that the median is not the same thing as the mean. The median is simply the middle value in a group of data and cannot tell you much about the rest of your data sample.

How do you calculate the median?

You find the median simply by sorting your data and selecting the middle observation. If you have an even number of data observations, there is no natural middle data point, so you must calculate the median by averaging the two middle observations. Mentally calculating the median is easy if your data set is limited, but for large data sets, you may want to look to Excel for assistance (see Figure 4.2).

Figure 4.2 — **Calculating the median**

The following instructions will help you calculate and display the median, as well as many more descriptive statistics. You can follow these steps if you are trying to calculate any of the descriptive statistics that follow. Learn it once; use it many times!

1. Open the spreadsheet containing your data.

2. Select "Tools" from your menu bar, and click "Data Analysis."

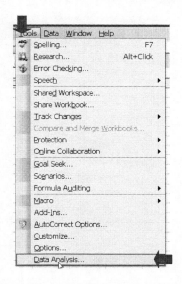

3. In the pop-up Data Analysis window, click "Descriptive Statistics" and then click "OK."

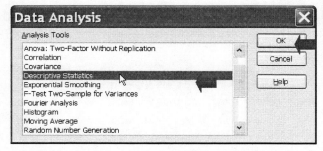

4. In the Descriptive Statistics dialog box, specify the range to analyze by highlighting the range of cells you want to analyze; include the column or row header where your data label is stored. The data range you highlighted will be entered into the range box.

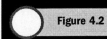

Figure 4.2 — **Calculating the median (cont.)**

5. Click "Labels in First Row" and click "Summary statistics." Then click "OK."

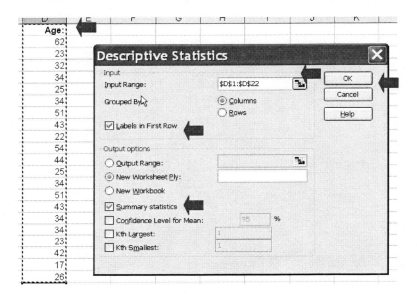

6. Excel will analyze the data and produce a summary chart on a new sheet within your workbook, summarizing several descriptive statistics including the median. Here you can see that 21 records were analyzed. The mean was 35.87, the median was 34, and the mode was 34.

	A	B
1	*Age:*	
2		
3	Mean	35.85714
4	Standard Error	2.636995
5	Median	34
6	Mode	34
7	Standard Deviation	12.08423
8	Sample Variance	146.0286
9	Kurtosis	-0.50881
10	Skewness	0.471656
11	Range	45
12	Minimum	17
13	Maximum	62
14	Sum	753
15	Count	21

Mode

What is the mode?

The mode is the most common value, or the value that occurs most frequently in your data set.

When is it appropriate to use the mode?

The mode is appropriate for all types of numbers (nominal, ordinal, interval, and ratio).

Extreme values in your data set do not affect the mode, but the mode can differ significantly from the mean if your data is skewed.

When is it inappropriate to use the mode?

Some sets of data do not have a mode. For example, there will be no mode if all the data values are unique. Furthermore, some modes are statistically meaningless. For example, knowing that most patients have 14 letters in their last name will not help you analyze patient fall data.

It is possible to have multiple modes if one or more values are listed the same number of times. Take, for example, a study of the ages of clients visiting your sports medicine clinic. If your data for one month showed three clients who were 31 years old and three clients who were 37 years old, you would have a distribution that is multimodal.

How do you calculate the mode?

To manually calculate the mode, sort your data from high to low (or vice versa) and then count the number of times each value occurs. The value that occurs most frequently is the mode.

For larger data sets, Figure 4.3 will take you through the process of calculating the mode using Excel.

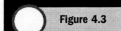

Figure 4.3   **Calculating the mode**

To calculate the mode in Excel, follow these steps:

1. Open the spreadsheet containing your data.

2. Select "Tools" from your menu bar. Click "Data Analysis."

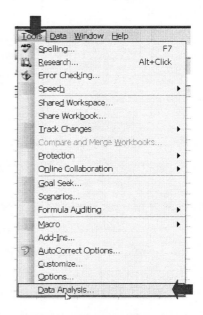

3. In the pop-up Data Analysis window, click "Descriptive Statistics," and then click "OK."

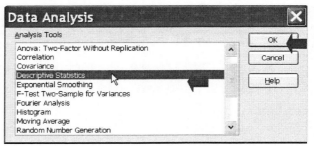

4. In the Descriptive Statistics dialog box, specify the range to analyze by highlighting the range of cells you want to analyze; include the column or row header where your data label is stored. The data range you highlighted will be entered into the range box.

5. Click "Labels in First Row" and then "Summary statistics." Then click "OK."

Figure 4.3 — Calculating the mode (cont.)

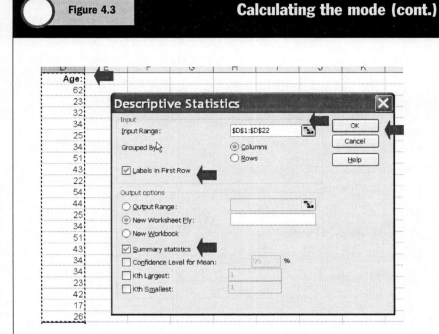

6. Excel will analyze the data and produce a summary chart on a new sheet within your workbook summarizing several descriptive statistics including the mode.

Here you see that 21 records were analyzed. The mean is 35.86, the median is 34, and the mode is 34.

	A	B
1	Age:	
2		
3	Mean	35.85714
4	Standard Error	2.636995
5	Median	34
6	Mode	34
7	Standard Deviation	12.08423
8	Sample Variance	146.0286
9	Kurtosis	-0.50881
10	Skewness	0.471656
11	Range	45
12	Minimum	17
13	Maximum	62
14	Sum	753
15	Count	21

Percentile and quartile

What are percentile and quartile?

Percentile analysis is a simple way to describe how a particular observation relates to the entire group. Using percentile you could, for example, determine how a physician's medical record delinquency rate or postsurgical infection rate compared with that of other physicians on staff.

Percentile charts are divided into tenths (percentages), and data is placed into these one-tenth segments accordingly.

Quartile analysis also shows how a specific observation relates to the group. However, quartile analysis divides data into four equal units, or quarters. Quartile analysis is useful when there are extreme outliers in your data—it effectively flattens out the data.

When is it appropriate to use percentile or quartile?

These analyses are useful for summarizing very large data sets, such as standardized test results in schools. If you scored in the 90th percentile, that means you scored better than 90 percent of the respondents and you scored in the top 10 percent of those taking the test.

When is it inappropriate to use percentile or quartile?

Analyses such as percentile or quartile will not be useful if your data is normally distributed and the values of the mean and the median are similar to each other.

How do you calculate percentile and quartile?

To calculate percentile or quartile manually, follow these steps:

1. Sort your data from high to low (or vice versa).

2. Count the number of rows of data and then add one.

3. Divide by 10 for percentile; divide by 4 for quartile.

   Statistics Basics, Global Edition

4. Take the resulting number and, starting in the first row, count up by that number, dividing the data each time you reach a break (at each tenth or quarter).

See Figure 4.4 for Excel instructions for creating percentile and quartile charts.

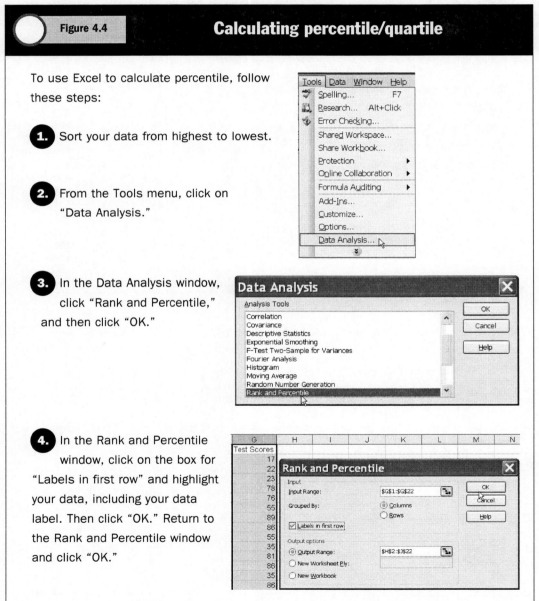

Figure 4.4   **Calculating percentile/quartile**

To use Excel to calculate percentile, follow these steps:

1. Sort your data from highest to lowest.

2. From the Tools menu, click on "Data Analysis."

3. In the Data Analysis window, click "Rank and Percentile," and then click "OK."

4. In the Rank and Percentile window, click on the box for "Labels in first row" and highlight your data, including your data label. Then click "OK." Return to the Rank and Percentile window and click "OK."

Figure 4.4 **Calculating percentile/quartile (cont.)**

5. The results of the rank and percentile analysis will be created in a new sheet in your spreadsheet that will resemble the example shown here. In this example, the three individuals who scored 86 were ranked third in the group, and this placed them in the top 20% of those taking the test, or better than 80% of the other individuals.

Point	Test Scores	Rank	Percent
18	98	1	100%
7	89	2	95%
8	86	3	80%
12	86	3	80%
14	86	3	80%
20	85	6	75%
11	81	7	70%
17	80	8	65%
4	78	9	60%
5	76	10	55%
16	75	11	50%
19	56	12	45%
6	55	13	35%
9	55	13	35%
21	45	15	30%
10	35	16	15%
13	35	16	15%
15	35	16	15%
3	23	19	10%
2	22	20	5%
1	17	21	0%

To use Excel to calculate quartile, follow these steps:

1. Open the spreadsheet that contains your data.

2. From the tools menu, click on "Insert Function."

3. In the Insert Function pop-up window, click on "Quartile," click "OK," and then follow the instructions in the wizard.

4. Excel will display values between 0 and 4, where 0 is the smallest number in the list, 1 represents the lowest quartile, or the bottom 25%, 2 represents the bottom 2 quartiles, or the bottom half, and so on.

The Excel wizard for instructions for median and mode will also automatically calculate the additional descriptive statistics shown in Figure 4.5.

Figure 4.5   **What Excel can do for descriptive statistics**

Statistic	Description
Standard deviation	The dispersion of the group of data values
Standard error	The square root of the sample size (n) divided by the standard deviation over the square root of the sample size (n)
Range	The difference between the largest and smallest values
Minimum/ maximum	The smallest and largest values in your data set
Sum	A total of all the values in your data set
Count	The number of observations or values in your data set
Skewness	The degree of symmetry in the distribution around a central axis
Confidence level	How much your value deviates from the mean

To download a customizable version of this form or other figures from this book, go to *www.hcpro.com/global* and click on "Tools."

Measures of variation (or dispersion)

Variation is normal and expected in all statistical processes, and understanding variation is fundamental in quality improvement efforts. You'd expect wait times and postsurgical infection rates to vary from patient to patient, month to month, and institution to institution. In the healthcare industry, we assume that outcomes in patient care are the result of the process of delivering care. Many hands and many departments are involved in even the simplest of tasks—for example, giving a patient a medication. Outcomes are a result of interconnected processes, and variation is to be expected.

Process improvement can be accomplished once you understand the process and the types of variation in it, and you can implement changes to further reduce variation or to improve the part of the process that affects the outcome.

Variation is the amount of spread or dispersion in the data. Two common measures of variation are used in statistics: range and standard deviation.

Range

What is range?

The range is the difference, or spread, between the largest and smallest values in your set of observations.

When is it appropriate to use range?

Range displays the widest possible spread of your data. For example, the range of refrigerator temperatures recorded in the blood bank is an important statistic. Range is also commonly displayed in stock market quotes and other situations in which it can provide some perspective on a given value (e.g., today's stock price) in relation to others (e.g., the 52-week high and low prices for the same stock).

When is it inappropriate to use range?

Range will not be a very useful measurement if your data has extreme outliers—observations of data points that are significantly farther out from the central value than the other observations in the set. Outliers may be either higher or lower than the mean and do not convey quality or lack thereof; they simply mark a significant aberration in the data.

For example, the range of patients' height in a primary care clinic where you have ages ranging from infant to adult would probably yield meaningless information.

How do you calculate range?

To calculate range, follow these steps:

1. Sort your data.

2. Select the largest value and the smallest value in the data set.

3. Subtract the smallest value from the largest value. The result is your range.

Standard deviation

The use of standard deviation in quality improvement efforts was a concept borrowed from the manufacturing industry in the Total Quality Management movement. In the process of manufacturing an automobile, there are tens of thousands of individual parts. Each part needs to be made to precise specifications, and a failure in any of these parts could result in a costly recall of vehicles. This limits or controls are set that specify the acceptable level of variation in the manufactured parts.

In this example, to reduce variation around the mean, or to reduce the number of parts that fall outside the preset level of variation, is to increase the quality of the automobile. So the manufacturer may strive to reduce the frequency of parts defects to a level in which deviation is occurring at a standard of less than 1 percent of the time.

In healthcare, standard deviation and statistical process control are applied in a similar way.

We know that the processes in the provision of quality healthcare are complex, and that multiple processes and people are necessary to accomplish seemingly simple things, such as administering antibiotics to a patient with pneumonia.

We also understand from industry research that the time it takes to provide the first dose of antibiotics affects the patient's recovery and length of stay.

So use of a core measure such as "patients receiving antibiotics within four hours of arrival," is seeking to:

- Measure the timing of the first dose

- Ensure that virtually all patients get their antibiotic within that time frame

- Ensure that the variation in first-dose time does not swing wildly around that goal

It is not acceptable for most patients to receive antibiotics within three and a half hours, and for every eighth patient to receive antibiotics eight hours from the time of arrival. In this example, descriptive statistics of mean, median, and mode would not be adequate to judge the quality of your process. You might have a mean time within four hours because the majority of patients receive the antibiotic within three and a half hours, but the random patients who wait eight hours will not be detected using descriptive statistics analysis.

We know that these outliers are significant to the outcome of the patient, so we have to look to measures of variation and standard deviation to assess the process. In this process, these random patients fall out of the control limits, and as a result, they are put at risk. This is an example of a process that has statistical outliers and needs analysis and improvement efforts.

What is standard deviation?

As described earlier, standard deviation is a powerful statistical measure of the variation or dispersion of data around the mean, or average, value. The larger the standard deviation, the wider the dispersion around the mean.

When is it appropriate to use standard deviation?

Standard deviation is a frequently used statistic in all businesses and research settings to measure the spread of data distribution. You use all data points when calculating standard deviation, whereas the range considers only the highest and lowest values in the set.

Standard deviation helps you determine where the majority of your data points should fall. It also highlights patterns of data that could be caused by a special variation, rather than normal variation. Special patterns, such as the outlier administration of antibiotics in the earlier example, can call attention to areas that need improvement.

Standard deviation is almost always applicable to your statistics projects. When you calculate a standard deviation, you get a measurement or a value, and the unit of measurement is always the same as the unit of measurement in the sample data. For example, if you are calculating standard deviation for infant weights in kilograms, the unit of measure for the standard deviation will also be in kilograms.

A word about statistical process control

As mentioned earlier, special patterns of data can be cause for concern. These patterns are actually statistical rules that identify special cause variation, and as a group, they are referred to as statistical process control.

To determine whether a process is statistically "in control," you can plot your data, calculate mean and standard deviation on a run or line chart, and apply statistical process control rules to the chart. This type of chart is called a control chart, and the rules you employ are called statistical process control rules. We'll discuss these in more detail shortly.

How do you calculate standard deviation?

Calculating standard deviation is more easily done by computer (see Figure 4.6) or calculator than by hand, although it can be done manually. Fundamentally, standard deviation is the square root of the variance of a set of data. The variance is calculated by squaring each observation's deviation from the mean and then calculating the average of all the squared deviations. This text will not suggest that you learn how to manually calculate standard deviation with paper and pencil. It is more important to understand the concept of standard deviation and its many uses. However, if you wish to learn the mathematical formulas for calculating standard deviation, please see the resources in the Appendix at the end of this book.

For now, it is assumed that you have access to a calculator with a standard deviation function or a spreadsheet or statistical software package that can calculate it for you.

 Statistics Basics, Global Edition

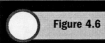 **Calculating standard deviation**

To calculate standard deviation in Excel, follow these steps:

1. Open the spreadsheet containing your data.

2. Select Tools from the menu bar and click "Data Analysis."

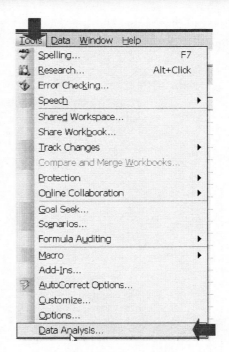

3. In the pop-up Data Analysis window, click "Descriptive Statistics" and then click "OK."

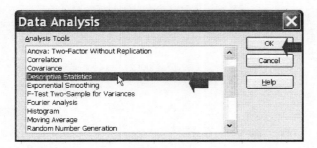

4. In the Descriptive Statistics dialog box, specify the range to analyze by highlighting the range of cells you want to analyze; include the column or row header where your data label is stored. The data range you highlighted will be entered for you into the range box.

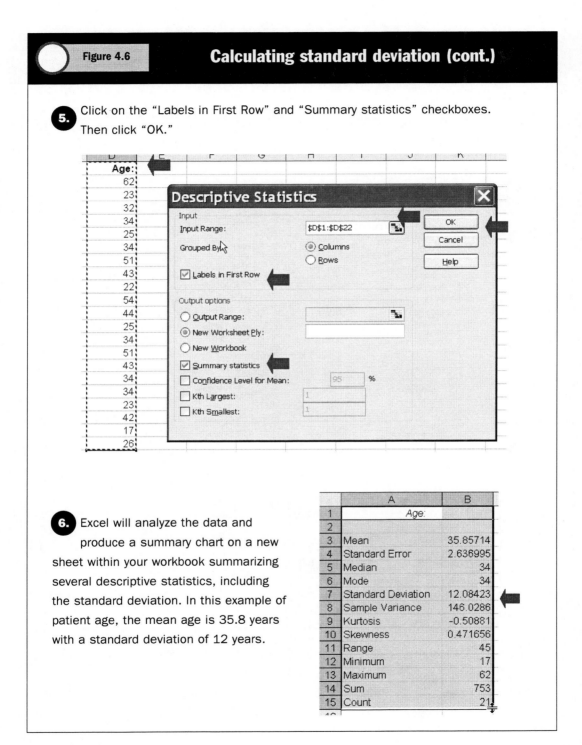

Figure 4.6 — **Calculating standard deviation (cont.)**

5. Click on the "Labels in First Row" and "Summary statistics" checkboxes. Then click "OK."

6. Excel will analyze the data and produce a summary chart on a new sheet within your workbook summarizing several descriptive statistics, including the standard deviation. In this example of patient age, the mean age is 35.8 years with a standard deviation of 12 years.

	A	B
1	Age:	
2		
3	Mean	35.85714
4	Standard Error	2.636995
5	Median	34
6	Mode	34
7	Standard Deviation	12.08423
8	Sample Variance	146.0286
9	Kurtosis	-0.50881
10	Skewness	0.471656
11	Range	45
12	Minimum	17
13	Maximum	62
14	Sum	753
15	Count	21

 Statistics Basics, Global Edition

Control chart

What is a control chart?

Control charts display the variation in a process over time and are used to distinguish between normal process variation and process variation resulting from special causes. Control charts also illustrate process stability or instability over time.

For each time period reported on your graph, a control chart displays the data value, a center line (usually the mean), and upper and lower **control limits.** Control limits are levels or lines on a control chart that mark the upper and lower limits within which all plotted points should lie if the process is in control.

Control limits are traditionally set to plus or minus three standard deviations of the center line. The control limit that is set to three standard deviations above the center line is called the upper control limit (UCL). The control limit that is set to three standard deviations below the center line is the lower control limit (LCL). If three standard deviations below the center line result in negative numbers, the LCL is set at zero.

Control charts are useful in quality improvement efforts because they help you assess the stability of a process over time. However, it's important to understand that a control chart can tell you whether a process is in control, but it says nothing about the quality of that process. If, for example, you have a consistently high infection rate, month after month, year after year, you have a bad process that is in control.

The chance of an observation being outside the three-standard-deviation control limit is about 1 percent: One case in 100 will fall outside three standard deviations. The data points that fall outside of the control limit represent something that needs further investigation—it could be an indicator of good data, but it could also be an indicator of bad data.

When is it appropriate to use a control chart?

You can use control charts if you have at least 12 to 18 months' worth of data or units of data—in other words, control charts are most useful if you have a lot of data/observations.

Control charts identify the following:

- **Common cause variation:** This is a natural, expected variation that occurs within all processes. Generally, you can reduce this type of variation only by changing the process itself. This is one major goal of quality improvement efforts.

- **Special cause variation:** This is an outlier that results from an unexpected but explainable change in the process. For example, in a measure of patients receiving printed discharge instructions, a special cause variation would be if you received the printed discharge instructions one month late.

Distinguishing between special and common cause variation is critical in your improvement efforts. Plotting your data and the standard deviation on a control chart can help you distinguish between the two types of variation.

There are many types of control charts. The selection of one control chart over another is based on the type of data/the type of measure/sample size. Figure 4.7 displays some more common types of control charts.

Figure 4.7 | **Types of control charts**

Type of control chart	Chart selection requirements
P-chart	Most useful with processes that are measured by the proportion of occurrences over the entire sample at risk. The data is often attribute data, or data that is counted as unique events, such as deaths, falls, or infections. Used with large sample sizes.
U-chart	Also called rate charts and used with ratio-type outcome measures. In a U-chart, control limits are calculated for each time period on your chart. The data is often attribute data. Used with variable sample sizes.
M-chart	Used with continuous variables and large sample sizes.
MR-chart	Used with continuous variables and small sample sizes.
X-bar and R-chart	Useful for small sample sizes (less than 10) with variable data (data measured on a continuous scale, such as time, temperature, etc.).
X-bar and s-chart	Useful for larger sample sizes (greater than 10) with variable data.

To download a customizable version of this form or other figures from this book, go to *www.hcpro.com/global* and click on "Tools."

Statistical process control rules

A process is considered "out of control" if it fails one or more of the basic statistical process control rules. Listed are three common tests to identify special cause variation:

- One or more data points falls above or below the three-standard-deviation control limits:

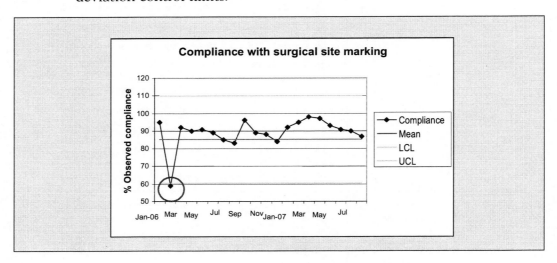

- There is a sequence of eight consecutive data points on one side of the center line:

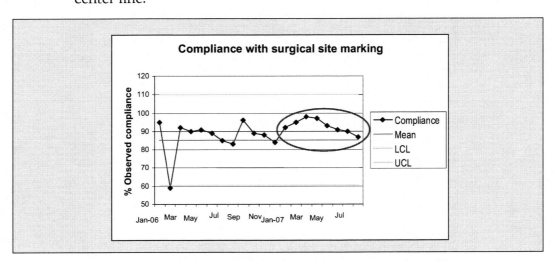

Statistics Basics, Global Edition

- There is a series of six consecutive data points steadily increasing or decreasing:

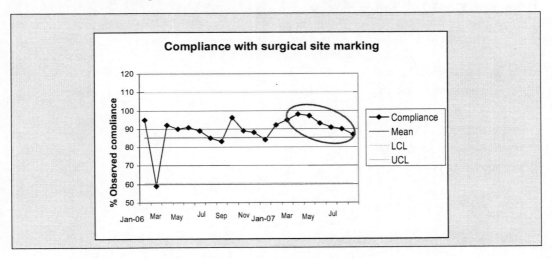

How do you create a control chart?

Creating a control chart is a matter of calculating the mean and standard deviation and plotting them in a line chart. Figure 4.8 shows the basic steps for creating a control chart in Excel.

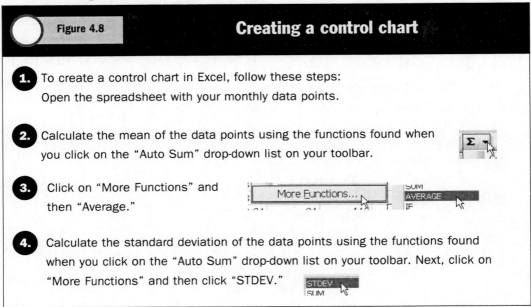

Figure 4.8 — **Creating a control chart**

1. To create a control chart in Excel, follow these steps:
Open the spreadsheet with your monthly data points.

2. Calculate the mean of the data points using the functions found when you click on the "Auto Sum" drop-down list on your toolbar.

3. Click on "More Functions" and then "Average."

4. Calculate the standard deviation of the data points using the functions found when you click on the "Auto Sum" drop-down list on your toolbar. Next, click on "More Functions" and then click "STDEV."

Figure 4.8 | **Creating a control chart (cont.)**

	A	B	C
2	Month	*Compliance*	Mean
3	Jan-06	95	85.34
4	Feb	59	85.34
5	Mar	92	85.34
6	Apr	90	85.34
7	May	91	85.34
8	Jun	89	85.34
9	Jul	85	85.34
10	Aug	83	85.34
11	Sep	96	85.34
12	Oct	89	85.34
13	Nov	88	85.34
14	Dec	84	85.34
15	Jan-07	92	85.34
16	Feb	95	85.34
17	Mar	98	85.34
18	Apr	97	85.34
19	May	93	85.34
20	Jun	91	85.34
21	Jul	90	85.34
22	Aug	87	85.34
23	Stand Dev	8.24	
24	Mean:	85.34	

5. After calculating the mean and standard deviation of your data, enter the mean in your spreadsheet next to each monthly data point.

6. Next, you will need to calculate your UCL and LCL. To determine your LCL, multiply your standard deviation by three and subtract that value from your mean. Then add that same value to the mean to get your UCL. Enter your UCL and LCL into your spreadsheet.

7. Finally, chart the values in the spreadsheet, including the monthly data, the mean, and both the UCL and LCL. Use the line chart for your chart type.

	A	B	C	D	E
2	Month	*Compliance*	Mean	LCL	UCL
3	Jan-06	95	85.34	61	110
4	Feb	59	85.34	61	110
5	Mar	92	85.34	61	110
6	Apr	90	85.34	61	110
7	May	91	85.34	61	110
8	Jun	89	85.34	61	110
9	Jul	85	85.34	61	110
10	Aug	83	85.34	61	110
11	Sep	96	85.34	61	110
12	Oct	89	85.34	61	110
13	Nov	88	85.34	61	110
14	Dec	84	85.34	61	110
15	Jan-07	92	85.34	61	110
16	Feb	95	85.34	61	110
17	Mar	98	85.34	61	110
18	Apr	97	85.34	61	110
19	May	93	85.34	61	110
20	Jun	91	85.34	61	110
21	Jul	90	85.34	61	110
22	Aug	87	85.34	61	110
23	Stand Dev	8.24			
24	Mean:	85.34			

Statistics Basics, Global Edition

Controlling trouble

It is important to remember when applying statistical process control rules to a control chart that an outlier does not necessarily mean trouble. Both positive and negative outliers exist: If your mortality rate were an outlier on the low side, you would have a reason to celebrate. However, an outlier can be the result of bad or missing data, an issue that you will need to investigate, identify, and resolve.

If you do have negative outliers that do not result from bad data, read on. The reason for negative outliers must be investigated in some depth, and you will learn about some tools to accomplish this in Chapter 5.

Taking it to the next level

Know when to seek help. If you need to calculate more-sophisticated control charts, you may need to use one of the many statistical process software packages available. Another alternative to developing the expertise internally for advanced statistical analysis is to contact the statistics department of your local college or university. Graduate students are sometimes available to assist in your analysis.

Drawing conclusions and planning next steps

What is included in this chapter:

- Understanding variation

  - Brainstorming
  - Flow charts
  - Cause and effect diagrams

- Improvement

  - Generate ideas
  - Report findings, recommendations
  - Continue to measure

So you found something. Maybe your data isn't telling the whole story, or your results are skewed. Now what?

You have planned and completed your study, and you have aggregated and analyzed your results. You have performed one or more statistical tests on the data, compared yourself to benchmarks, spread the data around the standard deviation, or studied one of the many tests of variability. Maybe you have plotted your data on a control chart and identified areas where your data is considered out of control.

Fear not: The hardest parts are behind you, and you don't have to start all over again. We are in the final phase of the statistical process cycle: the phase of drawing conclusions, reporting results, and planning next steps.

Perhaps your facility originally picked the area of study because it was high-volume, high-risk, or particularly problem-prone. Let's assume at this point that you have determined that your process met one of the statistical process control rules for being out of control. You now are at the step of discovering where the problem is in the process and what to do next (see Figure 5.1).

Analyze the cause of the problem. Armed with the information you have collected and prepared up to this point, you now move into the more familiar process improvement steps. Your goal is to understand the process and uncover the cause of the special cause variation. You will have several suggested tools that you may use to assess your process and several designed to help you improve your process.

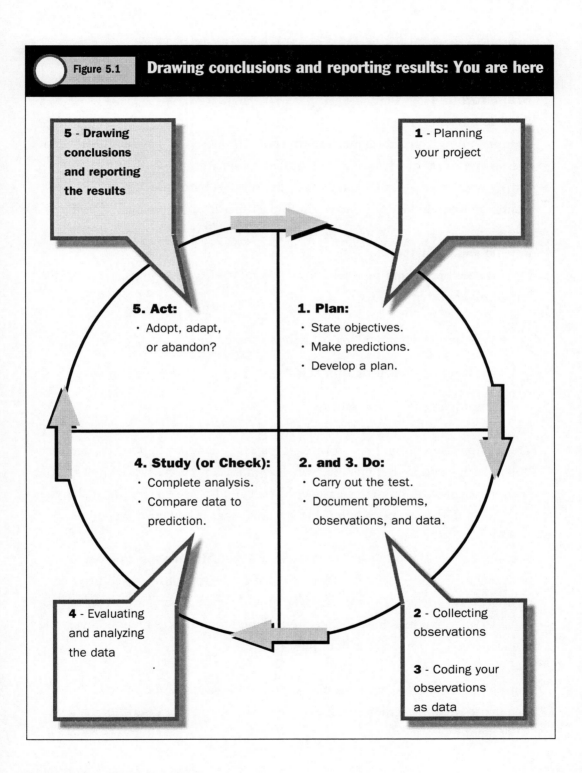

Figure 5.1 Drawing conclusions and reporting results: You are here

5 - Drawing conclusions and reporting the results

1 - Planning your project

5. Act:
- Adopt, adapt, or abandon?

1. Plan:
- State objectives.
- Make predictions.
- Develop a plan.

4. Study (or Check):
- Complete analysis.
- Compare data to prediction.

2. and 3. Do:
- Carry out the test.
- Document problems, observations, and data.

4 - Evaluating and analyzing the data

2 - Collecting observations

3 - Coding your observations as data

Understanding variations and implementing improvements

Brainstorming
What is brainstorming?
Brainstorming is a performance improvement tool used to generate ideas about the process or problem you have identified. Brainstorming is done in a group setting with attendees who have expertise in the subject under investigation. Brainstorming can be done once or multiple times in an improvement initiative.

How do you brainstorm?
You can use brainstorming to carry out several critical next steps, including identifying:

- All the steps that you are studying in the process

- Problems in the current process

- Improvements to the process

The composition of the brainstorming group is paramount to good outcomes. You need the actual staff members who are most familiar with the process, at both manager and non-manager levels. You will also need a facilitator charged with keeping the process moving and ensuring that it remains productive.

A common pitfall in brainstorming sessions, especially in a mixed group of both managers and staff, is hesitancy by staff to identify problems in front of managers. A skilled facilitator can overcome this by encouraging all participants to offer opinions in sequence around the room. In this manner, everyone is encouraged to voice his or her opinion.

During brainstorming, there should be no debate or discussion of any idea mentioned by a group member. There will be time for discussion at subsequent meetings.

When brainstorming, the facilitator simply records all comments on flip charts or uses some other means that's visible to all, and keeps the group focused on the task at hand.

Prior to the group convening, all group members should receive an agenda of what is to be accomplished during the meeting, the location and time of the meeting, and a list of other participants. Normally, the facilitator would distribute meeting materials, unless the group is lucky enough to have both a team leader and a facilitator—in this case, the team leader would normally be responsible.

In addition to receiving an agenda, members should receive a packet of information about the project that will allow them to become familiar with the subject prior to attending the meeting.

Things you may want to include in the information packet are:

- The charts and graphs you prepared

- A copy of the original presentation

- The timeline you made for management describing the study

- Any other relevant documents

Following the brainstorming session, the facilitator must ensure that the material presented at the meeting is sent in hard-copy form to all participants in preparation for any further involvement in the project.

Creating a flow chart

What is a flow chart?

A flow chart is a graphical display of the steps in a process. You can use it to understand the current process, identify areas of weakness in the process, and recommend process improvements to minimize the problems you identify in the current process. Creating flow charts is a useful and necessary step.

How do you create a flow chart?

When creating a flow chart, your first step is to identify the specific process you are trying to flow. Make sure it is of a manageable size and scope—you may need to have multiple process flows for a measurement you are studying. This would be preferable to a process flow that goes on forever.

Next, use the brainstorming strategy to identify the activities and decision points in the process. Low-tech visual aids can assist in this step. For example, cover the walls of a room with deli paper or large flip chart paper to allow the group members to flow the process. You can also use small sticky notes to record steps in the process. This has the advantage of allowing you to move the notes around the flip chart paper as you refine your process flow.

Basic flow charts display all processes as rectangles, and decision points in the process as diamonds (see Figure 5.2). The direction of the flow is depicted using arrows to connect the boxes and diamonds.

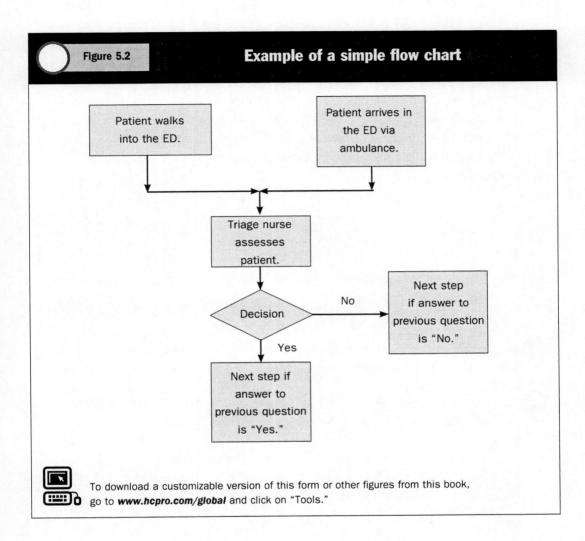

Figure 5.2

Example of a simple flow chart

To download a customizable version of this form or other figures from this book, go to *www.hcpro.com/global* and click on "Tools."

Following are tips for creating a basic flow chart.

1. You can create basic flow charts in Microsoft Word, by using the Drawing toolbar and the text boxes to enter the words. To display the Drawing toolbar in Word right-click on a blank space in your normal toolbar and then click on "Drawing."

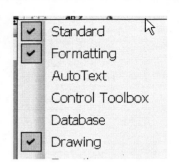

2. The Drawing toolbar will display in either the upper or the lower part of your screen.

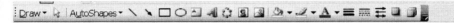

3. To add flow chart shapes, click on "AutoShapes" on your Drawing toolbar, click the shape you want, and then click where you want to draw the flow chart shape.

4. To add connectors between the shapes, click on "AutoShapes" and then click on "Connectors." Select the connector line you want.

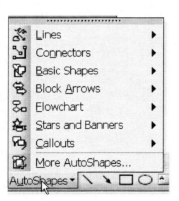
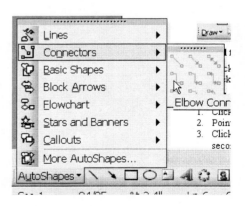

5. Point to where you want to lock the connector, and then click the first connection site you want. Point to the other shape, and then click the second connection site.

Creating a cause-and-effect diagram (also called a fishbone diagram)
What is a cause-and-effect diagram?
Cause-and-effect diagrams generated by brainstorming are a useful tool for identifying and organizing possible causes of a problem.

How do I create a cause-and-effect diagram?
You can create a cause-and-effect diagram by identifying the problem you want to investigate further on the right side of your paper. From the left, you begin drawing the "fish bones" that are the major causes of the identified problem.

Major causes are often identified under categories such as:

- People

- Procedures

- Policies

- Equipment and materials

As you identify more levels of detail under each broad category, you can begin to construct the smaller bones of the fish (see Figure 5.3).

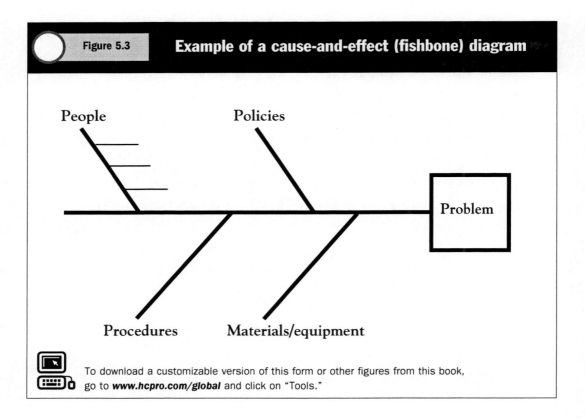

Figure 5.3 — **Example of a cause-and-effect (fishbone) diagram**

To download a customizable version of this form or other figures from this book, go to **www.hcpro.com/global** and click on "Tools."

Generating improvement ideas

Once you have flow-charted your process and dissected the possible causes for the problem you discovered, you and your team have the necessary tools to generate improvement ideas. This is the step in which you formulate recommendations for improving steps in the process.

These suggestions should be supported by evidence wherever possible. Brainstorming is an effective tool in this step of the process.

Reporting findings and recommendations

The final step in the statistical cycle is the generation and presentation of your final report. The final report will generally consist of both a written and an oral presentation to the leadership and the process owners. Materials prepared for your final report should include:

- Your original problem statement

- Your data analysis

- Graphical displays (charts)

- The process flow

- The cause-and-effect diagram

- Your recommendations for improving the process

Continuing to measure and report on the process

. . . And the process begins anew!

Following approval of recommended improvements, you jump back onto the process improvement cycle in the Plan phase. Once you've figured out where the problem is and how you are going to fix it, you implement your improvement initiative and continue to collect data on the process.

It is important to continue data collection to ensure that your improvement initiative has had its desired effect and actually improved your outcomes. But don't get discouraged by the thought of not being finished: It is tremendously satisfying to see statistical evidence indicating that you have made a difference in the quality of the healthcare delivered to your patients—after all, isn't that why we got into healthcare to begin with? Continued data collection and analysis is the way to ensure continued improvement in the future.

Conclusion

Planning, collecting, and reporting statistics can be challenging, especially if you've never done anything like this before. However, once you've become familiar with the terms and methods used in statistics processes, you can apply them to future quality improvement projects and other initiatives. And with your hospital under increasing pressure to show results, to demonstrate compliance, and to provide comparison data, the time has never been better to hone your statistics skills—or at least to proceed without fear.

Use the resources available to you, and seek successful projects in healthcare facilities that are similar to yours. A huge amount of statistical information is available online, but you may have equally valuable expertise in-house. Enlist help and support from your coworkers.

Don't be afraid to make mistakes and learn from them, and be sure to save and share your data, analysis, and results whenever possible. When you've proven your ability to gather and present meaningful statistics, others might look to you as a process improvement expert!

See the Appendix on the following pages for additional sources of information about statistics in healthcare.

Additional resources

If you've completed a statistics-intensive project and discovered that you're more numbers-oriented than you thought, perhaps it's time to seek more advanced knowledge.

You have plenty of options.

If your facility is located near a business school, college, or university, contact the mathematics or outreach department and see whether personnel or programs are available to help you take your knowledge of statistics to the next level.

In addition, consult other hospitals in your area. If the healthcare facility across town is working on or has completed a statistics-based performance improvement initiative, people there may be willing to discuss what works and what doesn't. One of the keys to any successful data-gathering and analysis project is to collect as much knowledge as you can before you start. Other hospitals may have ideas that can help you get buy-in from your team and leaders, streamline your processes, simplify your data gathering, or avoid mistakes before they occur.

Publications

A variety of publications expand on the basic concepts discussed in this book. Check your local library, college library, or bookstore. Following is a selection of books that may help you. (This list is not intended to be all-inclusive.)

For information about The Joint Commission's statistics expectations, check out these titles from Joint Commission Resources, Inc. (U.S.A.):

- *A Pocket Guide to Using Performance Improvement Tools in Health Care Settings*, Third Edition, 2006

- *Managing Performance Measurement Data in Health Care*, 2001

For more general help with statistics, consult these resources:

- *Basic Skills in Statistics: A Guide for Healthcare Professionals*, by Adrian Cook Gopalakrishnan Netuveli, and Aziz Sheikh © 2003 Class Health, Scotland.

- *Making Sense of Statistics in Healthcare*, by Anna Hart © 2001 Radcliffe Publishing Ltd., Britain.

- *Business Statistics Demystified*, by Steven M. Kemp, PhD, and Sid Kemp, PMP © 2004, McGraw Hill Cos., U.S.A.

- *Even You Can Learn Statistics: A Guide for Everyone Who Has Ever Been Afraid of Statistics*, by David M. Levine and David F. Stephan. © 2005, Pearson Prentice Hall, U.S.A.

- *Introductory Statistics, Fifth Edition*, by Prem S. Mann. © 2004 John Wiley & Sons, Inc., U.S.A.

For Excel-specific statistics help:

- *Evidence-Based Statistics Workbook* by Jennifer Peat © 2008 Blackwell Publishing, Britain.

- *Excel Data Analysis: Your Visual Blueprint for Creating and Analyzing Data, Charts and PivotTables*, 2nd Edition, by Jinjer Simon © 2005 John Wiley & Sons, Inc., U.S.A.

- *Statistics for Health Policy and Administration Using Microsoft Excel* by James E. Veney © 2003 Jossey-Bass Inc., U.S.A.

Journals

Peer-reviewed journals that have very good resources for quality and patient safety statistics include the following:

- *Health Care Statistics*, from the BMJ Publishing Group Ltd., subsidiary of the British Medical Association (Britain).

- National Association for Healthcare Quality's *Journal for Healthcare Quality* (U.S.A.).

- *Nurse Researcher: The International Journal of Research Methodology in Nursing and Health Care*. A research journal written specifically for nurses and healthcare staff members. This journal is for research specialists, clinicians, students and aspiring researchers and includes international features. Published quarterly by RCN Publishing Co., London, England.

- PubMed (*www.pubmed.gov*) is a service of the U.S. National Library of Medicine and includes more than 16 million citations from Medline and other life science journals for biomedical articles dating back to the 1950s. PubMed includes links to full-text articles and related resources. **Note:** You will need access to a medical library and its subscriptions to access the full content of some articles.

Online resources

The following Web sites will help you hone your statistics-gathering skills, and provide useful data or demonstrate best practices in collecting meaningful statistics. The following organizations provide a variety of data collection and reporting information and other statistical resources for hospitals and healthcare systems. This list is not all-inclusive.

- **Agency for Healthcare Research and Quality (AHRQ)** *www.ahrq.gov*: The U.S. government's AHRQ Web site has an extensive data collection, including the Quality Indicators and Patient Safety Indicators (*www.qualityindicators.ahrq.gov*), the Healthcare Cost and Utilization Project database (*www.ahrq.gov/data/hcup*), and other public information.

- **AHRQ Culture Survey** *www.ahrq.gov/qual/hospculture*: This Web site provides a validated survey of U.S. hospital patient safety culture, including some empiric data. It also offers a reliable data-collection tool and suggestions for use in trending performance over time.

- **Australian Council on Healthcare Standards (ACHS)** *www.achs.org.au*: Established in 1974, the ACHS is an independent, non-profit organization with the goal of improving health care quality in Australia through continual review of performance, assessment, and accreditation. The ACHS is the principal independent authority on measurement and implementation of quality improvement systems for Australian healthcare organizations.

In 2005, the ACHS established **ACHS International (ACHSI)** for international accreditation. ACHSI standards are based on ACHS standards; elements can be modified to ensure that standards are culturally appropriate for countries and cultures, while remaining comparable to the standards used in healthcare organizations in Australia. The ACHS and ACHSI are accredited by The International Accreditation Program of the International Society for Quality in Health Care (ISQua).

The "Research" area of the ACHS Web site may be of particular interest to those interested in gathering and interpreting statistics.

- **Canadian Council on Health Services Accreditation (CCHSA)** *www.cchsa.ca*: A national, nonprofit, independent organization that provides national and international healthcare facilities with voluntary, external peer review to assess the quality of their services. The CCHSA standards include core set of performance measures, and some statistical knowledge is required for accredited organizations' continuous improvement efforts. The "Leading Practices" area of the CCHSA Web site highlights innovative, process-based activities that healthcare facilities have developed related to CCHSA's quality standards.

- **CCHSA International:** The CCHSA's international branch adapts the CCHSA's Client-Centered Approach accreditation standards for international clients.

CCHSA and CCHSA International are accredited by ISQua.

- **Centers for Disease Control and Prevention's National Center for Healthcare Statistics (NCHS)** *www.cdc.gov/nchs*: This U.S.-based site provides statistics and reports on a wide range of topics. Tools include surveys and data-collection systems, as well as online forums devoted to nationwide healthcare initiatives, data collection, and ambulatory care branch statistics, among others.

- **Health Quality Service (HQS)** *www.hqs.org.uk*: The HQS (Britain) is the longest established health accreditation service in Europe. The HQS works with UK and international healthcare organizations to improve the quality of patient care through consultancy services and the development of healthcare standards and assessment processes.

- **HQS International** standards are based on the HQS standards used in Britain and include some statistical requirements. More information can be found at the International Programmes area of the HQS Web site.

  The HQS is part of CHKS Ltd. **CHKS Group**'s Healthcare Accreditation and Quality Unit (*www.chks.co.uk*) is an independent provider of healthcare information and data analysis tools and services. CHKS uses statistical data to boost healthcare organizations' efforts to improve care. The CHKS Web site includes examples of the importance of statistical data in healthcare improvement, and success stories from hospitals.

- **Institute for Healthcare Improvement (IHI)** *www.ihi.org/ihi/results*: IHI is a nonprofit organization based in the U.S.A. devoted to applying effective quality improvement strategies to healthcare. The site includes extensive resources, including collaboratives, literature, and data collection and analysis tools. It offers evidence-based process information and some data for comparative purposes, as well as access to collaboratives. The Improvement Methods section of the IHI Web page includes downloadable tools in a variety of computer formats for data collection, reporting, and statistical analysis. The IHI's Workspace area can be used to track improvement projects and collected data. Information about a variety of healthcare improvement initiatives worldwide is also available.

- **The International Quality Indicator Project® (IQIP)**
  www.internationalqip.com: This project assists healthcare organizations in identifying opportunities for improvement in patient care. Almost 180 healthcare organizations in 12 countries use the IQIP tools to collect, analyze, and compare clinical and administrative healthcare data. IQIP offers four sets of measures, called indicator sets, that focus on acute care (including hospital-based ambulatory care), psychiatric care (behavioral health), long-term care, and home healthcare. Participants select the appropriate indicator set, enter data monthly, and receive quarterly reports and links to relevant reports and reference materials. A computer with a color monitor is required, as well as software and training.

- **Institute for Safe Medication Practices (ISMP)** *www.ismp.org:* An authoritative source in the of best U.S.A. practices in medication safety, epidemiology, and incidence of errors with medication use. The ISMP also publishes a biweekly newsletter. This Web site includes a wealth of process recommendations and occasional evidence-based literature.

- **The International Society for Quality in Health Care (ISQua)**
  www.isqua.org: A nonprofit, independent organization based in Australia with members in more than 70 countries. ISQua provides services that help healthcare professionals and providers, researchers, agencies, and policymakers achieve excellence in healthcare delivery and continuously improve quality and safety of care. ISQua's clinical and other performance measures and indicators are consistent with worldwide trends toward measuring processes and outcomes that can lead to performance improvement.

- **The Joint Commission** *www.jointcommission.org:* The Joint Commission is the U.S.A.-based parent of the Joint Commission International. The Performance Measurement area of The Joint

Commission's Web site provides useful information about The Joint Commission's performance measurement initiatives, including meaningful, evidence-based performance measures, statistical approaches to data analysis, and identification of performance improvement and patient safety strategies. The Joint Commission also houses a growing comparative performance measurement database that healthcare organizations can use internally to help quality improvement activities and externally to aid accountability and advance research.

- **Joint Commission International (JCI)**
  www.jointcommissioninternational.org: This international arm of the U.S.-based Joint Commission offers a variety of statistics information as it relates to the JCI hospital accreditation program and International Patient Safety Goals. The JCI Center for Patient Safety area, sponsored by the World Health Organization, offers information about a variety of patient safety initiatives and quality measures.

  JCI is accredited by ISQua, the International Society for Quality in Health Care.

- **National Patient Safety Foundation** *www.npsf.org:* This site provides resources for patient safety and clinical care professionals in the U.S.A. (including a public list server) and provides patient/consumer/public education, leadership materials, and more.

- **National Quality Forum (NQF)** *www.qualityforum.org:* This membership group based in the U.S.A. develops and proposes national standards for quality and patient safety. The site includes a consensus statement on best practices for patient safety, as well as a consensus list of "never" events (serious reportable events) and recommendations for state-level reporting.

- **Quality Health New Zealand** *www.qualityhealth.org.nz:* Established by the New Zealand health sector to help improve the standards and performance of health and disability services, Quality Health New Zealand has provided assessment and quality improvement services in the health sector since 1990. This membership organization surveys public hospitals and health services, private surgical hospitals and clinics, continuing care hospitals, mental health services, and community health services. Quality Health New Zealand has strong links with The Joint Commission, the CCHSA, the United Kingdom Health Quality Service, and the ACHS.

- The **World Health Organization (WHO)** *www.who.int/features/ factfiles/health_statistics/en/index.html:* The WHO gathers information from member states, publications, and databases produced by its technical programs and regional offices to identify trends. Experts strive to produce accurate statistics for rich analysis of health information. The **WHO Statistical Information System (WHOSIS)** contains national statistics for 50 core indicators on mortality, morbidity, risk factors, service coverage, and health systems. WHOSIS' *World Health Statistics* compilation, presents the most recent health statistics for WHO's 193 member states. This compilation, available on the Web site, highlights 10 of the most important global health statistics for the past year, as well as an expanded core indicators set to 50 health statistics. All sections are available for download in Adobe PDF and Excel when applicable.

3